The Mind and Mood of Aging

The Mind and Mood of Aging

Mental Health Problems
of the Community Elderly
in New York and London

Barry Gurland
John Copeland
Judith Kuriansky
Michael Kelleher
Lawrence Sharpe
Laura Lee Dean

CROOM HELM
London and Canberra

The Haworth Press, Inc., 28 East 22 Street, New York,
New York 10010

British Library Cataloguing in Publication Data

The Mind and mood of aging.

    1. Aged, Mentally ill—Services for—Great Britain
    I. Gurland, Barry
    362.2′0880565   HV689

    ISBN 0-7099-1164-5

Published outside the Americas and the Philippines by Croom
Helm Ltd, Provident House, Burrell Row, Beckenham, Kent,
BR3 1AT, England.

Printed in the United States of America

Contents

List of Tables

Authors' Affiliations

Barry J. Gurland, M.R.C.P. (London), M.R.C. Psych.
Professor of Clinical Psychiatry
Director, Center for Geriatrics and Gerontology
Columbia University and
New York State Office of Mental Health
100 Haven Avenue
New York, New York 10032

John R. M. Copeland, M.A., M.D., F.R.C.P. (London), F.R.C. Psych.
Professor and Head of the University Department of Psychiatry
Director of the Institute of Human Aging
Royal Liverpool Hospital
P. O. Box 147
Liverpool L69 3BX
U. K.

Judith Kuriansky, Ph.D.
Clinical Psychologist
Center for Marital and Family Therapy
9 East 68th Street

Host, WABC Radio
1330 Avenue of the Americas

Specialty Reporter, WCBS-TV
524 West 57th Street
New York, New York

Michael J. Kelleher, M.D., M. Phil. (London), B.Sc. M.R.C. Psych.
Clinical Director
St. Anne's Clinic
Southern Health Board
Cork, Ireland

Lawrence Sharpe, M.B., B.S., M.R.C. Psych.
Assistant Professor of Clinical Psychiatry,
Columbia University
Research Psychiatrist,
New York State Psychiatric Institute
722 West 168th Street
New York, New York 10032

Laura Lee Dean, Ed.M.
Senior Staff Associate,
Center for Geriatrics and Gerontology
Columbia University and
New York State Office of Mental Health
100 Haven Avenue
New York, New York 10032

Foreword

The eventual outcome of a research endeavor is often difficult to foretell. Thus, the attempt to answer the simple question raised by Morton Kramer regarding the reported higher rate of schizophrenia in the U.S. than in the U.K. has led to a series of advances in knowledge which could hardly have been anticipated. The question came at a propitious moment. The present writer had made a series of visits to the various research centers in the United States, Europe, and Israel dealing with the biometric approach to psychopathology -- an approach which bases itself primarily on measurement and quantitative data. It soon became apparent that though similar terms were used cross-culturally to designate psychopathology, their meaning differed from country to country and even within the same country. A conference called for the purpose of resolving these differences under the auspices of the American Psychopathological Association and supported by the National Institute of Mental Health, failed to resolve the issues, though the discussions at the conference (<u>Field Studies in the Mental Disorders</u> (J. Zubin, Ed.)) achieved considerable progress. It also set in motion a plan for making a comparative study of the diagnoses in the United States and United Kingdom. At the same time, the plans for the World Health Organization Pilot Study in Schizophrenia began to be formulated. It became clear that both of these studies required new approaches for making cross cultural comparisons. This led to the development of new tools -- the semi-structured interviews -- which replaced the free wheeling clinical interviews used in the earlier studies as a basis for diagnosis. It also led to the utilization of a standard glossary in which the definitions of each diagnosis appeared. This eventually led to the development of the Research Diagnostic Criteria.

It was fortunate that when the need for the cross-cultural tools became apparent, the staff of the Biometrics Research Unit included several individuals who had already begun to develop systematic approaches to interviewing, especially Dr. Eugene I. Burdock and Dr. Anne S. Hardesty and Dr. Robert L. Spitzer, then a departmental fellow in training. They developed such instruments as the Ward Behavior Inventory, Mental Status Schedule, Psychiatric Status Schedule and a variety of others which provided items for the semi-structured interview to be used in the U.S.-U.K. Project together with the items selected from the Present State Examination Schedule prepared by John Wing and his associates at the Institutes of Psychiatry at the Maudsley Hospital in London, England.

It fell upon the shoulders of Dr. Barry Gurland to organize the initial project in the U.S.A. and for Dr. John Cooper to introduce it in the U.K.

The members of the cross-national teams in New York and London participated jointly in the preparation of the instruments to be used in the study, administered the interviews and engaged in the analysis of the data and the reporting of the results. It was truly a cooperative effort from beginning to end on the part of the entire staff but especially noteworthy were the contributions of Robert Kendell in the analysis of the data and of Larry Sharpe in the videotape studies.

In addition to the systematic approach to interviewing, several other new developments appeared. The staff introduced videotaping of interviews as a method for making comparative studies of diagnosis by exhibiting the videotaped interviews to groups of raters in geographically distant places. This project also demonstrated that despite cultural and social differences, objective cross-national comparisons could be carried out if sufficient care was taken in the preparation of the interview items and in the training of interviewers, systematic interchange of interviewers between the cities of New York and London, and collaboration between the administrative authorities of the two cities. In the wake of the many needs created by the cross-national study, improvements and new developments occurred in many interviewing and psychometric methods. These were, for example, in item construction, interview design (e.g., probes for determining whether a given line of inquiry is negative and can be discontinued), statistical techniques for assessing reliability and agreement between raters (e.g., Kappa), clustering methods, taxonomic analysis, etc. Many of these innovations came from the project staff in response to immediate problems of data analysis and others from collaborating consultants such as Dr. Jacob Cohen who developed Kappa, Dr. Joseph Fleiss who adapted it to further uses and Dr. Edwards Deming who provided the innovative sampling techniques.

One of the more ingenious innovations was the sampling strategy which developed a replicated design in which the whole sample consisted of five successive replications each of which was a random sample of the entire city. This not only provided a measure of internal consistency across the replications but also provided for the contingency that if funding were not continued, the results at any point would still be representative of the entire population.

It is a little difficult to realize that these innovations which now appear commonplace were not in existence when the U.S.-U.K. Project began. But the most unexpected development came with the extension of this primarily diagnostic effort into a deeper assessment not only of the mentally ill in the two cities but of the styles of life of the residents in the two cities with special reference to the overall well being of their citizens in health, health care systems, and the impact of the differences in the social, cultural milieu of the two cities. This expansion came after the initial study of the diagnostic project dealing with the age range of 20-59 came to an end and the geriatric study was begun. The machinery established for the original study was then applied to the problems of the elderly. After an initial assessment of patients in institutions (which again yielded no significant differences between the U.K. and the U.S.), it became clear that the majority of the mental health problems of the elderly inhered in the community; consequently, an assessment of the elderly in the community was undertaken. It became evident that it was impossible to isolate the diagnosis of mental illness from the matrix of the social-cultural-economic niche which the person occupied. Thus, a study of the ecological niche and the physical-social-cultural-economic milieu in which the niche was nested became essential.

The investigation focused on the needs of the individual under examination rather than on the needs of the service system which was trying to cope with his needs. Furthermore, in order to examine the problems of the elderly in depth, one assessment was not enough; successive follow-ups had to be undertaken to determine reliability and outcome in the light of the original assessment. Only in this way could the individuals vulnerable to mental disorders be identified and suitable intervention methods developed.

One of the more fruitful results of this endeavor has been the development of the Comprehensive Assessment and Referral Evaluation (CARE), covering the wide range of the mental and physical health and social conditions of the elderly as well as the services and supports they receive. It consists of 1500 items of information, an extensive set of global evaluations and a systematic narrative summary.

The full scope of the results can hardly be summarized here, but the fact that the elderly in the two cities are more alike than different, and the fact that despite the differences in the systems of care, much can be learned from the virtues and shortcomings of each, is quite apparent. Only by such comparative studies can improvements become possible.

From the initiation of the U.S.-U.K. Project beginning in 1963 it depended entirely on the efforts and cooperative spirit of the two teams -- one in the USA and the other in the UK. The story of how this cooperation developed despite initial differences in outlook, culture and expectancies cannot be told here, but it is a paradigm of international cooperation which is truly remarkable.

One indication of a successful study is the fate of those who participated in it. Nearly all of them now occupy prestigious positions in the field of psychopathology. Holding the study together from the very beginning and in its transition through its various phases was Dr. Barry Gurland. He, together with Dr. John Copeland, have steadied the course of the present project. They and their staff's scholarship, clinical acumen and research know-how have provided the continued leadership for this cross-national venture. Only those with the deepest compassion for the sufferings of the elderly ill could have persevered against the odds presented by this new undertaking. Following the project reported here, the collaboration with London has continued to the present day with Dr. Anthony Mann and now Dr. Alastair MacDonald leading the London team under the overall direction of Professor Michael Shepherd.

The most pressing question that still seems to face the elderly is the question of prevention of future disability. While the inroads of aging on life can not be avoided indefinitely, the quality of life can be much improved if we could determine beforehand those who are vulnerable to disorders of the senium. If they could be identified, perhaps therapeutic or preventive intervention could be introduced. Now that the descriptive phase of the work with the elderly is accomplished, it might be well to turn to the questions of etiology and vulnerability.

Joseph Zubin

Acknowledgments

Members of the United States-United Kingdom Cross-National Project who took part in the Geriatric Community Study are:

United States Project Staff: B. Gurland (U.S. Director and Principal Investigator),

L. Sharpe, R. Simon, J. Kuriansky, L. Dean, P. Stiller, R. Bennett, D. Wilder, J. Teresi, R. Golden, R. Gurland and D. Cook.

United Kingdom Project Staff: J.R.M. Copeland (U.K. Director and Co-Principal Investigator),

M.L. Robinson, R. Parker, A. Smith, A. Mann, Y. Tsegos and B. Robinson.

Consultants: J. Zubin (International Advisor), the late A. Goldfarb, W.E. Deming, J. Fleiss, M. Kramer and F. Post.

Collaborating Colleagues: G. Duckworth, P. Birkett, D. Cowan, and R. Paguni.

Project staff in New York are or were members of the Center for Geriatrics and Gerontology of the Faculty of Medicine of Columbia University and of the New York State Office of Mental Health; or of the Department of Geriatric Research, New York State Psychiatric Institute.

Project staff in London are or were members of the Department of Psychiatry, London University and of the Institute of Psychiatry at the Maudsley Hospital.

This study was funded mainly by grants from the National Institute of Mental Health (Grant No. 5R1MH09191), the Administration on Aging (Grant No. 93-P-57467), by the New York State Office of Mental Health, and the Department of Health and Social Security, London.

Prologue

The United States - United Kingdom Cross-National Project is an ongoing collaborative effort of two multidisciplinary groups based in New York at the Center for Geriatrics and Gerontology of the Faculty of Medicine of Columbia University and of New York State Office of Mental Health, and in London at the Institute of Psychiatry of London University. These groups have conducted an uninterrupted series of studies, beginning in 1965, directed at cross-national epidemiological and health service comparisons. The early studies were restricted to diagnostic issues with respect to adult psychiatric inpatients. These studies evolved into the geriatric age range, into the community, and into methods of comprehensive assessment addressing the distribution, nature and treatment of psychiatric problems in the context of the person's other health and social problems and the physical and social environment.

This monograph reports the principal methods and findings of the U.S.-U.K. Cross-National Geriatric Community Study. Although this report can be understood by itself, it is preferably read in conjunction with companion papers published by these investigators and their colleagues on this study (1-24), on other of the Cross-National Project's studies (25-40), and on the topics of depression, dementia and disability in the elderly (41-65). In order to keep this monograph as short as reasonable, the emphasis has been placed on a straightforward though fairly detailed presentation and interpretation of the study data. More complex analyses and the relation of the findings to other of the Cross-National Project's work or to the works of others has been more fully addressed in the companion papers cited above.

Section I
Overview

1. AIMS AND PURPOSES OF THE CROSS-NATIONAL GERIATRIC
   COMMUNITY STUDY

There are three principal aims in this cross-national
study (1). The first is to examine cross-national
differences among the community elderly in the prevalence of
psychiatric problems and their relationship to other health
and social problems; this aim is intended to increase the
understanding of the nature of psychiatric problems in old
age. The second aim is to examine cross-national differences
in the health care of aged persons, with a view to providing a
framework for improvement of health and support services to
those elderly with psychiatric problems who reside in the
community. The third aim concerns cross-national differences
in the course and outcome of psychiatric disability with
implications for the role of health care and community
resources in reducing chronic disability or its consequences.

The study includes the examination of two randomly
drawn probability samples of persons (445 in New York and 396
in London) over the age of sixty-five years and resident in
the cities of New York and Greater London. The people studied
were reinterviewed after one year in order to record their
use of health services and the course of their symptoms, or
the development of new symptoms. Social and medical factors
were studied in relation to psychopathological conditions.

2. CROSS-NATIONAL CONTEXT

A. Studies of the Prevalence of Psychiatric Problems among
   the Elderly in the Community

Kramer points out that although

> a considerable number of community surveys have
> been carried out in different parts of the
> world to determine the prevalence and, in a few
> instances, the incidence of mental disorders in
> the non-institutional population, the rates

1

reported in these studies do not lend
themselves to precise comparisons because of
differences in the underlying purposes of each
survey (66).

These purposes, in turn, required different definitions of a
case of mental disorder, and different case finding
techniques, diagnostic categories and data analysis methods.

The need for a prevalence study operated by
collaborative research teams working in more than one country
and using the same methods and diagnostic criteria in each
motivated this study. Leighton's Stirling County and Yoruba
comparison went some of the way toward achieving these ends
(67). This study goes further toward forming a basis for
testing hypotheses relating psychiatric problems to
cross-national variables and generating new hypotheses in
these areas.

At the end of a previous study by the U.S.-U.K.
Cross-National Project it was concluded that in examining the
cross-national variation in psychopathology

> London and New York would be an ideal pair of
> 'cultures' to compare . . . they are
> sufficiently similar in most of their social
> characteristics not to pose too many
> methodological difficulties, and yet they
> differ sharply in several important ways -- in
> the incidence of other forms of deviant
> behavior, in social attitudes to
> self-assertive and aggressive behavior, in the
> distribution of wealth and social attitudes to
> wealth, and in religious and ethnic composition
> (40).

In addition, these cities differ in the organization of their
health and social services for the elderly.

B.   Contrasts In Systems Of Health Care For Elderly
      Community Residents

An important aspect of this study is a comparison of
two health care systems with different perspectives. There
are well-known studies that have developed appropriate
methods to evaluate the prevalence of health needs and the
use of services among the elderly (68-69) but there has not
until now been the opportunity to compare in depth the
assessment and outcome of persons treated in two different
nations with contrasting but outstanding types of health
services. The National Health Service in the U.K. is a
universal compulsory prepaid scheme (private facilities are
available only on a small scale), organized in Regional Area

Health Authorities, supported by a wide range of local authority social services, and pivoting around the general practitioner and sometimes the social worker as the usual point of entry into the system; with the health care professionals generally being paid by central or local government salary or on a per capita basis. In the U.S. there are not one but several important systems, including the private and public sectors and various voluntary prepaid schemes; and payment is usually by a fee for service. The points of entry to the U.S. systems are various: the general practitioner or the specialist, public or private agencies, or an institution. The community services for the elderly appear to be more extensively developed and more systematized in England than in the U.S.A. (70-72). Not that either country has a monopoly on any particular service, but rather that services are more widely spread in England with centralized planning, organization and ongoing review being carried out on a national scale.

However, it is not sufficient to point to differences between the U.S. and the U.K. in services to the elderly without also considering whether the needs of the elderly differ in the two countries. Hoenig and Hamilton (73) have shown that the services required for the elderly in certain regions of England would not have been appropriate in another region they also examined. Thus, any study comparing health systems between the two countries must refer to the needs of the older people themselves.

C.   Need for Service Delivery for Elderly Community Residents

Both in England and the United States, observers have pointed to the need for improving the services to the aged in the community (68, 74-76). The elderly suffer from definite psychiatric symptoms in high proportion, perhaps 20 percent, of the general population over age sixty-five (74, 78-81). Their psychiatric symptoms are often accompanied by physical illnesses and they are often disabled by their symptoms (82-83). Yet the use of psychiatric outpatient services by the elderly is low (75), and less than 5 percent of this age group reside in institutions (84-85). It therefore appears that there may be many older people in the community who need psychiatric help, but do not receive it. These figures, supported by clinical experience, underline the importance of examining the delivery of community health and social services to the older person with psychiatric symptoms.

Systems of health care have generally evolved on a model more suitable for a younger, more assertive, vigorous and affluent age group, whose disorders tend to be more consistent with traditional organization of professional and specialist services. The elderly, however, are often financially hard-pressed and may be unable to afford expensive services or medicines (86). They may be physically immobile and unable to make the journey to outpatient settings. Their complaints often do not fit neatly into the compartments (such as "psychiatric," "medical" or "social" specialties) which are generally built into a health care system. They are often unaware of how to make the system work even when resources are available through the proper channels. They are sometimes confronted by the prejudice that psychiatric conditions in the elderly are irremediable, and by the low value attached to supportive rather than curative treatment (87). The present study is designed to keep in mind the needs of the elderly rather than the needs of the health care system.

3.   FEATURES OF THE STUDY

A.   Systematic Needs Assessment

This study is greatly facilitated by the use of semistructured interview techniques for health and social needs assessment in which the questions to be asked of all subjects are scripted and each of the relevant responses is defined. In this way we gain control over much of the variability due to differences between interviewers in style of delivery and in interpretation of responses. In addition, the responses of the subject to individual questions can be coded and analyzed independently of global impressions and diagnoses. Another advantage obtained from the use of semistructured interview techniques is that persons with similar symptom levels and patterns, but in different countries or different treatment modalities, can be identified and compared. For example, one can identify persons in the community who are similar in symptom patterns and severity to patients examined in hospitals or other institutions. The discovery of such people clearly raises important questions about the social factors determining institutional treatment.

B.   Follow-Up Assessment

A follow-up period of one year is included in the study in order to allow observation of changes in the severity of health and social problems; of ability to maintain independent function in the community; and the emergence of new symptoms. The initial assessment and the follow-up allows groups which are vulnerable to decline or loss of community tenure to be identified. Cross-national differences in these respects can lead to hypotheses concerning the relative therapeutic effectiveness of the health resources in the two countries. Knowledge about

vulnerable groups can considerably help in the planning for
efficient deployment of preventive services.

Another advantage to be obtained from the follow-up is
that differences in chronicity of mental or physical problems
between the two cities can be taken into account in
interpreting any differences in prevalence.

An important aspect of the follow-up study is the
oportunity to study the outcome of subjects with mild memory
impairments and other minor or early psychiatric symptoms.
These subjects constitute a high proportion of patients
attending general practitioners and are a challenge to
treatment which might prevent exacerbation of such minor
symptoms (88). Yet these conditions are difficult to
recognize and classify. Use of semi-structured interview
techniques and rating inventories for assessment allows the
assignment of a score of psychopathology within a wide range
of severity, so as to study persons with minor symptoms as
well as those with marked symptoms.

C.   Random Sampling

The choice of random (i.e., statistically random and
valid) samples of older people in the community offers
distinct advantages to the aims of this study. Estimation of
the prevalence of the associations, manifestations and course
of psychiatric problems is for the whole elderly community
and not restricted to those persons in contact with formal
health services (89).

The elderly living in the community is defined here as
those who are not living in institutional settings, such as
chronic disease hospitals, mental hospitals, nursing homes
(skilled nursing facilities), health-related facilities,
extended care facilities, adult homes or prisons. These
settings have their counterparts in both cities though the
above labels are more appropriate in New York while in London
the designations geriatric hospitals and local authority
homes correspond more or less with nursing homes and adult
homes respectively. The segment of the total elderly
population in institutional settings is approximately 5% in
both cities. For the purposes of this study the operational
definition of an elderly person living in the community was
that he lived in a dwelling unit in which there were less than
four unrelated persons mandatorily sharing a common dining
room. Thus at the boundary of this definition the elderly in
a single room occupancy hotel would be included unless the
only option for eating was to share a dining room with four or
more unrelated persons.

D.   Representing the Whole Elderly Population

The characteristics of the population that remains in the community can be influenced by the differential patterns of admission to institutions that exist in different communities and countries (75). A study by the U.S.-U.K. Cross-National Project, subsequent to the Community Study reported here, examined a representative sample of the elderly, aged sixty-five and older, in institutional settings in New York and London. The methods of assessment were compatible with those in the Community Study. The preliminary results of the Cross-National Geriatric Institutional Study have been reported elsewhere (25). When the community and institutional data are merged, it will be possible to construct a view of the health and social problems of a representative sample of the whole elderly population in these two cities.

Section II
Methods

1. ASSESSMENT OF HEALTH AND SOCIAL PROBLEMS AND SERVICE
    UTILIZATION

The assessment technique employed is a semistructured
interview, the Comprehensive Assessment and Referral
Evaluation (CARE), of proven reliability and validity, which
has been developed by this project (1). A full description of
the content of the CARE, its rationale and development, and
its reliability, is given elsewhere (4, 16-19). Only a brief
description of the CARE is given here, and an illustrative
segment of the interview is shown in Figure 2-1.

CARE interviews last from one to three hours,
potentially eliciting over 1,500 bits of itemized
information, an extensive set of global evaluations and a
systematic narrative summary. A modified version of the CARE
schedule is used for follow-up interviews.

The information collected by use of the CARE covers a
wide range of issues relating to the mental and physical
health and social condition of the older person, as well as to
services and supports received. These issues include
impairment of mobility and self-care, dependence on others
for personal services, formal treatment and medications
received, acute and chronic mental and medical illnesses
(e.g., heart disease, arthritis, dementia, depression, etc.),
malnutrition, housing difficulties, isolation, financial
hardship, and other social problems. The discrete bits of
information can be collapsed into scaled scores for each of
these issues. Rules are also provided for diagnostic
classification of acute and chronic mental and physical
illnesses and social problems. Global evaluations are made
of unfulfilled needs, severity of problems and of risk of
deteriorating or being institutionalized. Levels of stress
and positive health and assets are also assessed. A full list
of topic areas is shown in Table 2-1.

The key features of the CARE are its comprehensive and
systematic approach to the assessment of geriatric health and
social problems. In addition, it has the following

7

Figure 2-1. Illustrative Segment of CARE Interview

Question	Item	0	1	2	9
Have you had trouble sleeping over the past month? Have you been taking anything to help you sleep? (What?) Is there something that is interfering with your sleep? (What?)	Trouble falling or staying asleep	0	1	2	9
	Taking medication for sleep	0	1	2	9
If no trouble with sleep and not on night sedatives, skip to Q. 128.	Include any medication which the subject believes induces sleep or is actually sedative				
If on night sedatives, ask: If you weren't taking _____ would you have trouble sleeping? (What sort?)	Dependent on medication for sleep	0	1	2	9
If admits to sleeping difficulty or to taking night sedation: Do you have difficulty in falling asleep? Do you lie awake for long periods of time? (Waiting for sleep)?	Difficulty falling asleep	0	1	2	9
IF YES: (Does that bother you? How do you feel at those times? What goes through your mind? What keeps you awake?)	Sleep interrupted during night Include waking up after an initial cat nap and not being able to sleep again for some lengthy time	0	1	2	9
Is your sleep interrupted during the night?	Difficulty is due to altered moods or thoughts, or tension (e.g., lies awake with depressed or anxious feelings or thoughts)	0	1	2	9
IF YES: (What is the difficulty?) (What wakes you up?)					

Figure 2-1.

Question	Description			
(Any pain or discomfort?)	Difficulty, pain, malaise, itching, breathlessness, etc.	0	1	9
(Is it because you have to go to the bathroom?) (Can you get back to sleep after that?)	Wakes up (e.g., to empty bladder at night) but can go back to sleep thereafter	0	1	9
	No difficulty but seems to need less sleep	0	1	9
	Difficulty is noisy environment (rate also Q. 254)	0	1	9
Do you wake very early in the morning?	Awakes about 2 hours or more before normal time of awakening and cannot go back to sleep	0	1 2	9
IF YES: (Is that normal for you?) (What is your normal time?) (Can you get back to sleep?) When you get up in the morning do you feel you have had enough sleep? (Do you wake up feeling tired?)				
	Wakes up feeling tired	0	1 2	9
Do you sleep much during the day?	Sleeps for more than 2 hours during day	0	1 2	9
IF YES: For how long? How long do you sleep at night?	Sleeps more during day than at night	0	1 2	9
	DAY IS 8:00 A.M. TO 10:00 P.M.			

9

strengths. It draws on well-tried and tested scales within psychiatric, medical and social domains; the previous experience of the Cross-National Project in methods of assessing psychiatric disorders in hospitalized patients (40, 47, 53-55) has been the foundation for the psychiatric items in the CARE; both statistical and clinical methods have been used for selecting items, and extensive development took place based on actual experience with its use in the community, so that assessment is relevant to the problems found among community subjects and the special conditions of interviewing in that setting.

The arrangement of topic areas in the CARE reflects not only the comprehensive scope of the assessment, but also a tactful flow of the interview through the alternation of stressful topics (e.g., tests of dementia) with less stressful topics (e.g., physical health), and the ordering of topics so that they will make sense to the respondent rather than following only a professional logic (e.g., hearing impairment and auditory hallucinations are in linked sequence). In the interests of keeping the interview as short as possible, about half the questions in the CARE are contingent and need not be put to the respondent if a mandatory probe is negative. Finally, even if a respondent is unable to give valid answers to self report questions, there are test, observational and global items which can be completed.

Every effort has been made to include items which characterize mild as well as severe problems. For example, the section on depression identifies signs of fleeting depression, as well as the morbid qualities of the clinical depression. In order to avoid a confounding of the frequency of reported illness with the frequency of seeking medical treatment, the CARE includes details of symptoms rather than relying only on a diagnostic label known to the respondent. For example, the section on sleep disturbance has sufficient detail to allow a differential diagnosis to be applied to that symptom. The differential diagnosis of symptoms allowed by the CARE is crucial in the assessment of the community elderly; sleep disturbance, which in psychiatric hospital populations usually points to depression, in the community elderly must be evaluated not only for its psychiatric, but also for its medical and social implications.

All interviewing was completed by specially trained project personnel. In all the London cases and a random half of the New York cases the interviewer was a psychiatrist with a special interest in geriatrics. The remaining interviews in New York were by psychologists or social scientists. As described below the reliability within and between disciplines was good, especially for the psychiatric items.

The reliability of the psychiatric items in the CARE has been tested in several different ways.

(1)   In an early study, fully described elsewhere (58, 59), four raters (two psychiatrists and two social scientists) interviewed 8 elderly subjects drawn from the community.   Each rater interviewed 2 subjects and the remainder of the raters rated a videotape of the interview. The dementia score was based on 21 items and the depression score on 48 items.   Intraclass correlations (1 = project agreement and 0 = random agreement) were .82-.95 for dementia and .82-.97 for depression; there were no important differences between the ratings of the pairs of raters either within or between disciplines.

(2)   Another approach to assessing reliability was based on an analysis (α coefficient of Cronbach) of data gathered during the course of this study. The dementia score was again based on 21 items, but the depression score was based on 35 items. The coefficients for New York and London respectively were, for dementia .86 and .84; and for depression, .87 and .89 respectively.   There were no important cross-national differences.

(3)   During the course of the Cross-National Geriatric Community Study the psychiatrists based in New York and in London jointly rated a series of subjects, mostly in London but also in New York. Reliability for the psychiatric items was satisfactory and there were no important cross-national differences (17).

The reliability of the medical and social items was tested in the same several studies mentioned above and are reported with other characteristics of the homogeneous scales elsewhere (17). The alpha coefficients for the homogeneous scales are all above .70, the average value is above .80, and those for ambulation and activity limitation are both .95.

2.   SAMPLING DESIGN

A.   New York City

The sample used for our studies of New York City elderly was a probability sample that had been constructed by Lieberman Research, Inc. for a state-wide study of the elderly that they conducted for the New York State Office for the Aging in 1972. Segments of dwelling units already selected for New York City were used in this study. These segments are located in 66 clusters spread throughout New York City's five boroughs. This type of plan has two major advantages.

(1)   It provides, with computable ranges of
        reliability, estimates of characteristics of all
        individuals 65 years or older that reside in
        households in New York City, and

(2)   It provides an operational basis for statistical
        analysis and tests of hypotheses associated with
        the problems under consideration.

For our study we used a replicated design, by which the
whole sample is divided into five randomly selected,
stratified, inter-penetrating subsamples, in which each
household in New York City had a known chance of selection. A
major advantage of a sampling design that makes use of
subsamples is that it permits flexibility in the size of the
final sample without a commitment in advance to some definite
size. A rule of the procedure was to put into the field one
subsample at a time, and to put forth on it maximum efforts
before moving on to the next subsample. This procedure
ensures that the sample will not consist mainly of cases easy
to complete.

Another important advantage of the design in subsamples
is that each one provides an estimate of any characteristic
of the frame, wherefore comparison of the subsample estimates
for any characteristic provides, by a single calculation, the
standard error of any estimate that is calculated from the
whole sample (89).

As our sample was enumerated two years prior to our use
we found it necessary to up-date it. For this purpose records
of interviews were divided into two strata:

(1)   Dwelling units that in 1972 contributed an
        interview of someone in the household 65 years
        old or over.

(2)   Dwelling units where no one 65 years or over
        resided in 1972, someone over the age of 65 lived
        there before but was not interviewed, or there
        was no contact.

The appropriate sample to take from each stratum was
dictated by the statistical theory of optimum allocation of
effort to achieve the best precision possible for a given
cost (90).

B.   Greater London

There is often a choice between several frames that may
be used to cover a universe. For example, for this study in
London, the frame could have been portions of the Enumeration
Districts of London, similar to the procedure used for New

York. In the case of London, however, there was a simpler procedure, and that was to make use of the lists of community residents 65 years of age or over in possession of the general practitioners, to whom they are assigned for health care. Essentially all elderly persons living in a London community are represented on a general practitioner's list. Once arrangements were made for use of these lists, then a sample of individuals drawn from these lists led directly to a selected person by name and address. The sample in London, like the sample for New York, was laid out as a replicated design in subsamples.

The procedure used in London possesses the two advantages that are mentioned for New York. In addition, in London, the labor or preparation was made considerably less by use of names on the lists of general practitioners than it would have been by use of Enumeration Districts. In New York there were no lists available, so the sample was necessarily a sample of areas. A sample by use of either frame would give a valid unbiased estimate of what would be obtained by a complete coverage of the entire universe. A valid estimate is one for which one may compute an estimate of its standard error.

The advantages of drawing the sample in this way are clear. The principal disadvantage is that a doctor who has a large number of subjects in a sample may refuse to cooperate, in this case all those subjects are lost, fortunately rare. Doctors who were uncertain about helping were visited by Project members and the study explained in detail. Previous investigators agree that about 3% of old people are not on General Practitioners' lists (91). These are mainly vagrants who would not be found by a house to house survey and a small proportion of private patients who do not register with a National Health Service doctor. Most private patients register with both types of doctor.

There are instances in which one uses a combination of several kinds of frames. For a given size of sample in terms of patients, or of residents 65 years old or over in the community, the standard error of an estimate obtained by use of one frame will usually not be the same as the standard error that would be obtained by use of another frame, although use of either frame will give valid unbiased estimates.

In summary, it is only necessary that the totality of all sampling units in a frame shall cover the universe. A sample of sampling units drawn from any frame by any procedure for which the probability of selection of any given sampling unit is ascertainable, when combined with appropriate formulae of estimation, will give a valid estimate of the equal complete coverage. A further description of the sampling methods used in New York and London can be obtained from Dr. W. Edwards Deming.

3.   FIELD WORK METHODS AND RESPONSE RATE

Because of the differences in the way the samples were selected and because of environmental differences between the two cities, field work was carried out in a slightly different manner in New York and London (2).

A.   New York City

As discussed earlier, the New York sample was divided into two strata and each stratum required a different field work approach. Because each household in Stratum 1 had a member sixty-five years old or over in 1972, and because each of these individuals was interviewed at that time we had a list of their names, addresses and phone numbers. We sent a letter to each of these households, introducing our study, urging all household members 65 years old and over to participate (the Lieberman study had interviewed only one member), promising them confidentiality if they did participate, and notifying them that we would be in touch by telephone to arrange an appointment for the interview. In cases where letters were returned "addressee unknown, deceased, etc." a new letter was sent addressed to "Resident." A follow-up telephone call was made within a few days to arrange an appointment with the subject(s) and a randomly assigned interviewer. Interviewers were assigned to visit any household for which we had no phone number, or where there was no answer after numerous telephone calls had been made at different times of the day, and different days of the week. If no one was at home at the time of the visit we sent another letter to the household, informing them about our visit and requesting them to call our office so that we could arrange an appointment, or, if preferred, to return the enclosed stamped, self-addressed envelope and a card specifying a time convenient for an interview.

It was necessary to re-enumerate completely all selected households in Stratum 2. For this purpose we hired individuals, who were familiar with the cluster areas assigned them, to go to the designated addresses and take names from the mailboxes and building lists wherever available. We felt it desirable to mail the letters to a specific name rather than to the "Resident." After lists of these names and addresses had been compiled we sent a letter to each household explaining that an individual working with our organization, and possessing proper identification, would visit in the near future to ask a few preliminary questions about the household composition and to arrange for an

interview appointment with all members of the household age
65 and over.

These letters were followed in a few days by a visit to
the households by the independent field worker who enumerated
the households and made appointments with eligible subjects
whenever possible. Interview appointments were not always
easily scheduled. Subjects often postponed interviews,
hedged making appointments, or had misgivings about
participating.

A total of 445 interviews was completed in New York. In
order to get some of the interviews it was necessary to
schedule them outside of the subject's home. Some subjects
were afraid to allow strangers in, and others didn't want
anyone to see their living quarters. However, 396 (89%) of
the interviews were conducted in the subjects' homes, and
another 32 (7%) were conducted in the subjects' neighborhoods
(a building lobby, garden, senior center, or place of
employment). Only four (1%) were conducted in our offices,
and 13 (3%) were conducted by phone.

When there were two or more eligible subjects in a
single dwelling unit we arranged to send two interviewers
wherever possible so that the interviews could be conducted
concurrently. This was the most effective and tactful way of
keeping the subjects' interviews separate and independent of
each other.

New York City's elderly population is made up of many
ethnic groups and it was necessary to use an interpreter in 54
(12%) of the interviews. This includes one interview of a
deaf woman that was conducted with the aid of an interpreter
in sign language. In addition, a few of our subjects were
unable to answer questions due to such factors as organic
brain syndrome or coma. To include these cases in our
description of New York's elderly it was necessary to resort
to informant interviews in 26 cases (6%) of our sample. These
interviews were conducted with people who knew the subject
well. In 23 of the cases the informant lived with the subject
and in three cases the informant was a relative who lived
nearby.

Response Rate: Enumeration of 1,726 New York City
households (located in 66 cluster areas) yielded a total of
624 persons sixty-five years old or over. Of these 624
eligible subjects we were able to obtain information on 445
(a 71% response rate). Nine subjects who were eligible to be
interviewed either moved before an interview could be
arranged or were away from their residence during the entire
initial interview period. The remaining 170 subjects refused
outright to be interviewed, or gave so many excuses about

arranging a time and place that the interviewing period expired.

Table 2-2 shows the New York City response rate by Stratum and by Subsample.

B.   Greater London

London's sample of elderly was drawn from lists of general practitioners of whom some 3,000 serve London. These practitioners are divided into 11 areas, each controlled by an administrator, a registrar and a Family Practitioner's Committee. The general permission of the administrator for each area was obtained and the opinion on the feasibility of drawing the sample was obtained from each registrar. Each Family Practitioners' Committee was then approached separately with letters of introduction from the Department of Health and Social Security and the British Medical Association, which gave their permission for the sample to be drawn. We obtained a list of all the practitioners with patients in each area and sampled these at random. Letters were written to all the practitioners for their permission to see a sample of their patients. When this permission was obtained, we visited each of the 11 areas and sampled the practitioners' lists from a central register of patients over the age of sixty-five. Each subject was then written a letter enclosing an introductory letter from the doctor that explained the nature of the project and sought a time for interview. The endorsement of the study by the general practitioner was often influential in getting subjects to cooperate. However, one general practitioner, with a potential 19 subjects, refused to participate.

If subjects did not respond to correspondence, they were contacted by telephone, if they had one. Since 41% of the London sample are without telephones, it was necessary to visit many of the households to schedule an appointment. Nevertheless, interviewing subjects in London is clearly much easier than in New York. There are no areas of London where team members are afraid to go alone and elderly people appear willing to open their doors to strangers. Overall the Londoners would appear to be more cooperative subjects than New Yorkers; as evidenced by the higher response rate (81%), and by the fact that the research team was able to conduct all but one of the interviews in the subject's homes. Only 14 (4%) were informant interviews, and only three were interpreted.

Response Rate: A total of 644 individuals, sixty-five years old and over, were randomly selected from general practitioners' lists of patients in Greater London. Seventy of those drawn were ineligible for the study because they had moved away from the area, were confined to long-term institutions or were deceased. Of the 489 eligible subjects, 396 (81%) were interviewed. The remaining 93 potential subjects of our study either did not respond to correspondence, were never at home when called on, or declined to participate. Table 2-3 shows the London response rate by subsample.

C. Comparison of Difficulties Obtaining Interviews

Problems in getting interviews were more often noted by New York interviewers than by those in London. Table 2-4 shows that the New York team had trouble getting into a subject's home 11 times more often than did the London team.

D. Comparison of Difficulties in Conducting Interviews

In addition to getting subjects to agree to be interviewed and to gaining access to their homes, interviewers sometimes had difficulties in conducting interviews. The reasons for difficulties in conducting interviews have been grouped into a number of categories. The categories are as follows: (1) communication problems (both pathological and nonpathological), (2) inappropriate answers to questions, (3) difficulties in understanding the subject, and (4) response set biases. In all of these categories the interviewers working in New York City more often rated problem areas. It must be kept in mind that these problems are not mutually exclusive and some interviews were fraught with difficulties while most interviews were conducted smoothly without any problems.

The interviewers were asked to rate the following items if it was felt that any of them contributed to communication difficulties during the interview. The first group (Table 2-5) are nonpathological communication problems and the second group (Table 2-6) reflect pathology.

Nonpathological communication problems were indicated over three times more frequently in New York than in London; and pathological communication difficulties were nearly four times as frequent.

The interviewer was asked to rate the items shown in Table 2-7 if he felt that the subject had had difficulty in understanding the questions that were asked, and if he felt that this misunderstanding resulted in inappropriate answers to questions. The New York interviewers reported inappropriate responses twice as often as the London interviewers.

If the interviewer and/or the subject had difficulty in understanding each other due to language or other communication problem the interviewer rated another series of statements. See Table 2-8 for a comparison of these difficulties. The New York interviewers reported difficulty in understanding subjects three times as often as did the London team. However, in the majority of cases of communication difficulty in New York, the interviewers felt able, with perseverance, to understand the subject. In both cities there were only a few interviews where many or most answers could not be understood.

If an interviewer had doubts about the reliability of the data collected they were asked to rate what about the interview had caused these doubts. Table 2-9 shows the results. These items are not mutually exlcusive and since some interviews had more than one difficulty the numbers are not additive and do not total the number of interviews in which interviewers expressed doubt about the data. The frequencies of various response styles which caused raters to lack confidence in the data they collected are shown. Both New York and London interviewers rated doubts about their data most often being related to subject's tendency to say "no" to questions indiscriminately. This occurred in 11% of of New York cases and 5% of London cases. This response set was more than twice as frequent in New York as in London. The opposite response set tendency "exaggerating or saying yes indiscriminately" was rated more often in London than in New York (2% in London, but less than 1% in New York). Interviewers rated subjects as giving misleading answers about equally, 4% in both cities. Offhand replies and random answers were also noted almost equally (3% versus 2%) in New York and London.

Problems conducting interviews were much more frequently noted in New York than in London, and thus New York interviewers more often expressed not having complete confidence in the data that they collected. Table 2-10 exhibits this difference. New York interviewers had doubts about the data they collected more than twice as often as did the London interviewers, and this ratio was constant at every level of doubt.

In both cities we achieved satisfactory response rates (71% and 81%), which provide us with reasonable confidence in the representativeness of the samples and in estimating the prevalence rates of disorders. As you will see in Tables 3-2 and 3-3, the demographic profiles of the subjects interviewed are very similar to the profiles provided by the census data.

The New York interviewers did, however, express more difficulties in getting and conducting their interviews. Communication problems were more prevalent in New York. These communication disorders might have been misinterpreted as reflecting psychopathology, but because of the design of the CARE instrument which separates communication problems into two parts, it is apparent that most of the communication problems in interviewing were seen by the interviewers as nonpathological. It is the nonpathological communication problems where we see the biggest differences.

Table 2-1. A General List of the Topic Areas in CARE,
            In the Order in Which They Appear

Identifying data/Dementia I: (census type data)/country of origin/race/length of time spoken English

Dementia II: (error in length of residence/telephone number)

General inquiries about main problems

Worry/depression/suicide/self-depreciation

Elation

Anxiety/fear of going out/infrequency of excursions

Referential and paranoid ideas

Household arrangement/loneliness

Family and friendly relationships/current and past isolation index/closeness

Emergency assistance

Anger/family burden on subject

Obsessions/thought reading

Weight/appetite/digestion/difficulties in shopping and pre-paring food/dietary intake/alcohol intake

Sleep disturbance

Depersonalization

Dementia III: (Subjective and objective difficulty with memory/tests of recall)

(continues)

Table 2-1. continued

Fits and faints/autonomic functions/bowel and bladder

Slowness and anergia/restlessness

Self-rating of health

Fractures and operations/medical and non-medical attention/
    examinations/medicines or drugs/drug addiction

Arthritis/aches and pains

Breathlessness/smoking/heart disease/hypertension/chest pain/
    cough/hoarseness/fevers

Limitation in mobility/care of feet/limitation of exertion/
    simple tests of motor function

Sores, growth, discharges/strokes/hospitalization and bed-rest

Hearing/auditory hallucinations

Vision/visual hallucinations

Hypochondriasis

Disfigurement/antisocial behavior

Loss of interests/activities list

History of depression

Organizations and religion/educational and occupational history

Work and related problems/retirement history

Income/health insurance/medical and other expenses/handling
    of finances/shortages

(continues)

Table 2-1. continued

Housing facilities and related problems

Ability to dress/do chores/help needed or received

Neighborhood and crime

Overall self-rating of satisfaction/happiness

Insight

Mute/stuporous/abnormalities of speech

Additional observations of subject and environment/communica-
tion difficulties

Global ratings of severity, risk, fulfilled and unfulfilled
needs for psychiatric, medical and social problems
separately

Global ratings of distress, impaired performance, disturbance
to others and danger to self

Global ratings of nutritional risk

Global ratings of various psychiatric, medical and social
syndromes

Diagnoses of psychiatric, medical and social conditions

Global ratings of personal, physical and environmental assets

General stress scales

Systematic summary

Table 2-2. Response Rate by Stratum and Subsample
(New York City)

Stratum and Subsample	Households Screened N	Eligible for Study N	People Interviewed N	Response Rate %
Stratum I				
Subsample 1	91	74	52	70
Subsample 2	90	60	45	75
Subsample 3	90	59	46	78
Subsample 4	91	65	47	72
Subsample 5	90	57	45	79
Subtotal	452	315	235	75%
Stratum II				
Subsample 1	256	59	36	61
Subsample 2	257	68	50	74
Subsample 3	253	73	59	81
Subsample 4	252	57	34	60
Subsample 5	256	52	31	60
Subtotal	1274	309	210	68%
Both Strata				
Subsample 1	347	133	88	65
Subsample 2	347	128	95	74
Subsample 3	343	132	105	80
Subsample 4	343	122	81	66
Subsample 5	346	109	76	70
Total	1726	624	445	71%

Table 2-3. Response Rate by Subsample (Greater London)

Subsample	Selected from G.P. lists N	Not Traced or G.P. Refused N	Traced Ineligible N	Eligible for Study N	Interviewed N	Response Rate %
1	136	15	20	101	88	87
2	149	35	18	96	74	77
3	108	11	5	92	74	80
4	98	4	12	82	66	80
5	153	20	15	118	94	79
Total	644	85	70	489	396	81%

Table 2-4. Comparison of Obtaining Cooperation to Proceed
with Completed Interviews

Item Content	New York		London	
	N	(%)	N	(%)
Interviewer freely invited into home	345	(77%)	389	(98%)
Interviewed outside of the house before getting in	52	(12%)	4	(1%)
Interviewer had great difficulty getting in/or conducted interview outside of subject's home	48	(10%)	3	(1%)
Total Interviews	445	(100%)	396	(100%)

Table 2-5. Comparison of Non-pathological Communication
Problems

Item Content	New York N=445		London N=396	
	N	(%)	N	(%)
Foreign language	61	(14%)	7	(2%)
Unclear English dialect	2	(0%)	1	(0%)
Physical defect (speech disorder, deafness)	32	(7%)	15	(4%)
Low intelligence	2	(0%)	7	(2%)
Hostile, vague, muddled	41	(9%)	18	(4%)
Interview conditions unfavorable, distracting environment, relative, etc.	29	(7%)	1	(0%)
Total Non-pathological Communication Problems	167		49	

Table 2-6. Comparison of Pathological Communication Problems

Item Content	New York N=445		London N=396	
	N	(%)	N	(%)
Memory defect (clear-cut)	14	(3%)	7	(2%)
Memory defect (dubious)	9	(2%)	3	(1%)
Incoherent in clear conscious-ness, irrelevant or bizarre	4	(1%)	1	(0%)
Vividly pathological behavior (delusions, pressure of speech, gross suspiciousness)	6	(1%)	0	(0%)
Ambiguous pathological behavior (withdrawal, denial, distracta-bility)	21	(5%)	2	(0%)
Total Pathological Communication Problems	54		13	

Table 2-7. Comparison of Percentage of Interviews Where Subject's Responses Were Inappropriate

	New York (N=445)		London (N=396)	
	N	(%)	N	(%)
Subject gave inappropriate answers to:				
Some questions	15		5	
Many questions	3		3	
Most questions	1		1	
Total Interviews Where Subjects' Responses Were Inappropriate	19	(4%)	9	(2%)

Table 2-8. Comparison of Degree of Difficulty in Understanding Subject

	New York N	(%)	London N	(%)
Interviewer did not have difficulty understanding	380	(85%)	375	(95%)
Interviewer had difficulty understanding subject but:	65	(15%)	21	(5%)
Was able to understand with perseverance		44 (10%)		9 (2%)
Was unable to understand some answers		17 (4%)		7 (2%)
Was unable to understand many answers		1 (0)		3 (1%)
Was unable to understand most answers		3 (1)		2 (0)
Total Interviews	445	(100%)	396	(100%)

Table 2-9. Comparison of Reason(s) for Interviewers' Lack
of Confidence in Data Collected

	New York N=445		London N=396	
	N	(%)	N	(%)
Rater has doubts about data because subject:				
Exaggerates or tends to say yes, indiscriminately	2	(0%)	7	(2%)
Minimizes or tends to say no, indiscriminately	49	(11%)	19	(5%)
Gives misleading replies	26	(4%)	14	(4%)
Gives offhand replies or random answers	15	(3%)	8	(2%)

Table 2-10. Comparison of Interviewers' Confidence in Data Collected

	New York N (%)	London N (%)
Interviewer has reasonable confidence in data	317 (71%)	350 (88%)
Interviewer has doubts about data	128 (29%)	46 (12%)
Degree of Doubts		
A few doubts	78 (18%)	27 (7%)
Moderate doubts	40 (9%)	15 (4%)
Grave doubts	9 (2%)	4 (1%)
Data is worthless	1 (0%)	0 (0%)
Total Interviews	445 (100%)	396 (100%)

Section III
Results

1. COMPARISON OF DEMOGRAPHIC CHARACTERISTICS

A demographic description of the samples of aged people interviewed in New York and London is given in Table 3-1. The most important similarities and differences are discussed below.

The mean age of the New York elderly is the same as that in London -- seventy-four years for both cities. Similarly, the proportion of people who belong to the most vulnerable group of elderly, the "old old" (92), is much the same in the two cities, 40% in New York and 38% in London.

The age distribution of the females is similar in the two cities but for males there is a steeper decline in numbers after age eighty in London than in New York. Correspondingly there is a slightly higher female to male ratio in London than in New York. The fewer old men in London reflects the mortality of the World War I and of immigration that occurred just prior to the event (93). It is therefore not likely that the comparison of morbidity figures in the two cities will be appreciably influenced by differences in their age structure, but conditions that have an important sex difference will need to be analyzed separately for men and women; moreover, the cross-national comparison of conditions among the men will have to take into account the different age structure of men in the two cities.

The heterogeneous nature of the elderly population in the melting pot of New York City and the homogeneity of the elderly population found in London is shown in their racial and religious composition and their country of origin.

(1) Almost all the London elderly are white, while in New York 10% are black and another 10% of other origins. This contrast would be even more marked were it not for the fact that blacks have a shorter life expectancy than whites (94), and that Puerto Ricans are relatively new migrants to New York City and have not as yet brought with

them a proportionate number of aged relatives and have not as
yet aged themselves.

(2)   Again, in New York there is no religious group
which is dominant to the extent that the Church of England is
in London (where it accounts for 62% of the sample).

(3)   Most striking of all is the cross-national
contrast in the country of origin of the elderly. Fully 90%
of the elderly in London are native born, against less than
half in New York. One might expect then that the system of
care for the elderly in London is one which is well adapted to
them and relatively easy to apply in a uniform fashion
whereas in New York the system of care has no indigenous base
upon which to build and must instead respond to the changing
and varied cultural characteristics of the immigrants who
have become elderly, as well as to those who are native born.
On the other hand, it is possible that the New York elderly,
many of whom are pioneers and survivors as well as
adventurers, are better able to take advantage of whatever
services and resources are available to them than their
London counterparts. These background factors will acquire
meaning in the light of analyses to be presented on service
utilization.

The major categories of marital status (married and
widowed) show practically the same proportions in the two
cities. However, there are more divorced or separated
elderly in New York and more elderly that never married in
London than in the other city. The former figure is in line
with the generally higher divorce rate in the U.S. than the
U.K. (95-96). The latter figure reflects the unmarried women
in London who might have married if eligible men were not
killed in the war or did not emigrate.

Tables 3-2 and 3-3 compare New York and London sample
demographic characteristics with those of the entire
populations from which they were drawn. Because of the
similarity of the samples and census figures, it is
reassuring evidence that the samples are representative of
the two city populations.

Table 3-4 shows selected characteristics of the
life-style of elderly people in New York and London. These
characteristics are intended to present important
similarities and differences in the modal lifestyle of
elderly people in New York and London. About the same
proportion (within 4 percentage points) of the elderly in the
two cities live alone, do not have even one child living, and
have had no visitors in the past month. However, the London
elderly are more likely than the New York elderly to claim
that they have no confidante (20% versus 12%), and do not
belong to a club (60% vs. 49%) or a congregation (59% vs.

41%). These background characteristics will have a bearing
on our later analyses of the sources of informal support for
the frail elderly and those in crisis. They suggest that we
will find the sources of potential informal support are not
very different in the two cities, but perhaps with an edge in
favor of more readily available supports in New York than in
London.

There is a striking similarity between the two cities
in the proportion that spends little time in recreation (10%
or less) and in the distribution of the frequency of
excursions. About two-thirds of the elderly in each city get
out of doors at least once a day and only about 8% are
housebound. These figures give the first intimations that
the vigor and physical abilities of the elderly may be alike
in the two cities.

The selected items on crime, facilities, and housing
offer some indication of the quality of the environment in
which the elderly live in the two cities. Perhaps the most
telling indicator is that relating to rates of crime against
the elderly. Four times as many elderly in New York as in
London state that they have been attacked or their dwelling
burglarized in the previous year. However, in some material
ways the New Yorkers are better off in that they have
telephones, refrigerators and bathing facilities in their
dwelling units more often than do the Londoners.

About the same proportion (over a third) in the two
cities state that they live in a deteriorating neighborhood.
In either city, the elderly are likely to find themselves
stranded in areas which they once preferred but which have
changed in character to something less desirable. In both
cities the elderly are relatively stable residents; the
median number of years at the current address, 17 years in New
York and 15 years in London.

The space available in the dwelling unit has the same
median number of rooms in the two cities. However, the
majority of the New York elderly live in apartment houses,
whereas the two largest groups in London are about evenly
divided between apartment houses and one-family housing.

Apparently, there is no uniform superiority of one city
over the other in the social nexus of the elderly or in the
quality of their environment. We will later consider the
interaction of these social and environmental factors with
the elderly person's health status and morale. For the
present one can perhaps be impressed by the extent to which
social and environmental problems are shared by the elderly
in the two cities.

2.   COMPARISON OF HEALTH AND SOCIAL PROBLEMS

A.   Underline: General Note

The large amounts of data generated by this study make it desirable to have some way of summarizing the data for the purposes of cross-national comparisons. Two methods of data reduction are used: (1) scales based on previous work, our own and that of others, or on the face validity of items; and (2) scales based on empirical analysis of the body of data that we are reporting here. The first method has given rise to the "rational scales," the second to the "homogeneous scales" (17, 24). Each method has its virtues and drawbacks. Results on rational scales can be related to results of previous work and to conventional constructs from the clinical arena but may not be as valid or internally consistent when applied to the community elderly as they were in other populations. Homogeneous scales are, by reason of the manner in which they are derived, relatively comprehensive, internally consistent, and independent of each other (and are thus good summary data) when based on the data from the population on which they were derived, but may not serve equally well for constructs found useful in other related studies.

Following the general principles of our strategy for analysis, we make cross-national comparisons using both methods of data reduction (first the rational scales and then the homogeneous scales). We also compare cross-nationally the prevalence of individual items, including those which are the components of the scales. We place confidence mainly in results which converge on a given conclusion from all these methods of analysis.

The development of the rational scale and the psychometric properties and content of the homogeneous scales have been described elsewhere (17, 24). The content of the rational scales are given later in this section.

In the following analyses, we compare between the two cities the distribution of scores on the scales and the proportion of positive responses on the items. The purpose is to look for important differences or revealing similarities in terms of the stated aims of the study. In many instances, we provide the results of statistical tests to detect significant differences but we do this primarily because it has become usual to do so; we have serious doubts as to the usefulness of the information conveyed by the uncritical application of such tests to comparisons of survey data from two or more populations (97).

Finally, some mention should be made of our use of the Kolmogorov-Smirnov test (98) as one statistical test of significant difference. This test shows significant differences not only in means but also in the variance and shape of the distribution of scores. Thus the test may in some instances indicate a significant difference between the distributions of scale scores even where the means are identical. The test also compares the two observed cumulative relative frequency curves and is based on the largest absolute difference in the two curves. This value of the maximum difference in cumulative proportions is compared against a critical value derived from a mathematical probability model where it is assumed that the two distributions are identical.

B-1. Comparison of the Distribution of Scores on Rational Scales of Health and Social Problems

There are nine rational scales dealing with major areas of health and social problems and eight additional rational subscales of the major areas. The scales are listed in Table 3-5. The items making up the content of each scale are presented later in this section.

The means, standard deviations, and Kolmogorov-Smirnov test of the rational scales are shown in Table 3-5. In the subsequent tables each scale is reviewed and a table is provided giving the actual number of subjects at each score level and the cumulative frequencies for progressively lower levels and for progressively higher levels. Higher scores on a given scale indicate more, or more severe, symptoms or problems. Cumulative frequencies for progressively lower levels indicate the proportion of subjects scoring at a given level or worse; conversely, for progressively higher levels, the cumulative frequencies indicate the proportion at a given level or better. On the list of the items for each scale is given the percentage of subjects in New York and London who were rated as positive for that item (i.e., as having that characteristic).

The subscales are discussed separately at the end of this section but the cumulative tables for these scales are not presented here; they can be obtained from the authors (99).

Dementia. The mean score on the rational scale of dementia in New York (1.22) is almost twice as high as that in London (.67) and the Kolmogorov-Smirnov test is significant at the .01 level of confidence. The distribution of scores (Table 3-6) for New York lies above that of London (i.e., the scores in New York are higher than in London). There is also a longer tail (more very high scores) in New York than in London. For every level of score there are more subjects in New York than in London who score at that level or worse, the ratio being about 2 to 1 for almost every level. A score of 6 or more on dementia is particularly likely to be indicative of a severe clinical disorder; 5.8% of the New York elderly and only 2.5% of the London elderly score in this higher range. Furthermore, 1.6% of New York people score 12 or more, whereas none of the Londoners reach these highest (worst) scores.

The scale of dementia (Table 3-7) is composed mainly of errors in memory, orientation, and new learning, e.g., in identifying self and place; in reporting age, date and significant personal events; in learning the interviewer's name; and in recalling the names of famous persons. For 16 of the 22 items making up this scale, the population with that characteristic (i.e., making that error) is higher in New York than in London, for only four items is this relationship reversed and for two items the proportions are identical. Thus the higher mean and cumulative scores for dementia in New York compared with London arise from corresponding cross-national differences on the vast majority of items in the scale. The three exceptions (i.e., the London population higher than the New York population) include the two items dealing with knowledge of the president's or prime minister's name and this finding perhaps runs counter to the possibility that the worse scores in New York relative to London are a function of poorer education and more recency of immigration in New York than in London. One might expect more poorly educated and less well established residents in a country to have a worse, not better, knowledge of famous political figures.

Depression. The means for the scores on the rational scale of depression are remarkably similar (3.21 in New York and 3.17 in London), and the Kolmogorov-Smirnov test shows no significant differences between the distributions of scores on the two sides (Table 3-8). The cumulative frequencies of the distribution of scores on this scale indicate no difference of any importance between the New York and London elderly (Table 3-8).

The depression scale reflects all levels of severity of depression including demoralization or life dissatisfaction, vegetative signs of major affective disorder, psychotic symptoms, and suicidal impulses.

There are 38 items in all in this depression scale (Table 3-9), of which 8 do not reach a frequency of more than 2% in either New York or London and will therefore be disregarded in further discussion; those items represent the most intense levels of depression and, as expected, occur very infrequently in a non-hospitalized population. Of the remaining 30 items, 12 have higher frequencies in New York, 16 in London, and 2 are identical. Most of the differences between the two cities are small, but in 18 items there is a

50% or greater difference between the two sides with the higher proportion occurring in about equal numbers of items in the two cities. There may be some tendency for items that deal directly with the expression of depressed mood (e..g, worrying, crying, wishing to be dead, no enjoyment, not happy) to be more commonly rated as being present in New York than in London, whereas the converse may be true for items reflecting intrapunitive tension (e.g., self-depreciation, self-blame, irritability, withdrawal, difficulty relaxing and restlessness). However, on the whole there is no consistent cross-national difference that emerges from analysis of the rational scale of depression.

Total Physical Illness. The means for the rational scale of physical illness are practically the same in the two cities (5.11 in New York and 5.31 in London), and the Kolmogorov-Smirnov test reveals no significant differences in the distributions of scores on the two sides. Nevertheless, the cumulative scores show that a greater proportion of people in New York have lower (better) scores than people in London. The table (numbered 3-10) of cumulative frequencies clarifies that there is a difference in favor of better scores in New York but only at the lowest (best) ranges of scores (24.8% score 1 or better in New York vs. 16.7% in London). At most levels of scores the differences between New York and London are slight at the most.

The items in this scale (Table 3-11) cover a wide variety of self-reported symptoms with medical details related by the subject in response to probes put by the rater. A few symptoms measured by interviewer observations are also included. Topics include symptoms in the following areas: alimentary system, sleep disturbance, autonomic symptoms, disorders of consciousness, genito-urinary problems, arthritis and other aches and pains, symptoms of heart and respiratory disease, the early warning signs of cancer and the after-effects of advanced cancer, stroke, serious operations and fractures. There are 71 items in all, of which 26 do not occur more commonly than in 2% of the population in either New York or London. Of the remainder there are 21 items in which the proportion in London is greater than that in New York, and 21 where the converse holds, with three items having the same proportion of subjects rated positive in the two cities. Thirteen items show cross-national differences of 50% or more, with 5 being greater in New York and 8 in London. There may be a tendency for positive ratings on items reflecting respiratory complaints to predominate in London and possibly for symptoms of coronary heart disease to occur more commonly in New York. On the whole what differences emerge are those relating to types of symptoms rather than with respect to overall severity or number of symptoms.

Total Perceptual Impairment. The mean score on the rational scale of perceptual impairment is distinctly higher in London than in New York (2.19 vs. 1.53 respectively) and the Kolmogorov-Smirnov test is significant at the .01 level. The distribution of scores on this scale is generally higher (worse) in London than in New York (Table 3-12). This cross-national discrepancy is quite marked across the whole range of scores with the maximum relative difference being at scores of about 8 or higher, at which level the London proportion (9.3%) is almost twice that of the New York proportion (4.9%).

Items in this scale cover two major areas: hearing and visual difficulties. There are 21 items in all (Table 3-13). Fourteen of those items have higher proportions of positive responses (i.e., having that type of perceptual difficulty) in London and 4 in New York, with 3 being equal. Of the 14 items with predominance in London, 11 deal with hearing difficulty, while of the 4 items predominating in New York only 1 deals with hearing difficulty. Put another way, there are 12 items dealing with hearing difficulty and 11 of these show a predominance in London and only 1 in New York. Further reinforcement for these findings is obtained from focusing on the 11 items showing a cross-national discrepancy of 50% or more. Ten of these latter 11 items deal with hearing and 9 out of the 10 predominate in London. It can be concluded that a higher proportion of the elderly in London have hearing problems than the elderly in New York, though visual difficulties are no more common in one than in the other city.

Immobility. The mean scores on the rational score of immobility are almost identical in New York and London (2.68 and 2.69 respectively) and the Kolmogorov-Smirnov test shows no significant differences between the two cities. The cumulative frequencies of the distribution of scores on this scale show that there are no differences of any importance between the New York and London elderly (Table 3-14). If anything, there is a slight tendency for the New York elderly to have more low scores and also more high scores (i.e., more extreme scores) than the London elderly. Items in the scale reflect difficulty in self-care (basic and instrumental activities of daily living such as using the toilet or bath, preparing meals, shopping, and doing household chores); inability to perform physical activities; and a frail or ill appearance. These features represent the final common pathway of a variety of common chronic illnesses of old age.

There are 38 items in all in the rational scale of immobility (Table 3-15). In 11 instances the proportion of respondents with that item characteristic does not rise above 2% in either sample and will not be further discussed here. Of the remaining 27 items, 10 have higher proportions responding positively (i.e., having that characteristic) in

New York and 14 in London, while 3 have equal proportions in the two cities. In only 7 items are there cross-national differences of 50% or more in proportions of positive responses with 3 being predominant in New York and 4 in London. None of these differences suggests consistent cross-national differences of importance.

Inadequate Activities. The mean score on the rational scale of inadequate activities is higher in London (4.58) than in New York (3.81) and the Kolmogorov-Smirnov test is significant at the .01 level of confidence. The cumulative scores on this scale show that New York subjects, relative to London, have more very high (most inadequate) scores (5.4% to 3.5% have scores of 10 or higher), fewer scores in the middle ranges, and more low (least inadequate) scores (e.g., 54.6% to 36.4% have scores of 3 or less (Table 3-16). There is therefore a curvilinear relationship between the two cities in these cumulative scores.

The list of items in the scale of inadequate activities is concerned with non-participation in a fairly wide range of activities including excursions, social contacts, chores, recreation and attendance at organized meetings. There are 14 items in all (Table 3-17). Nine of these predominate in New York and five in London. Five items show a cross-national discrepancy of 50% or more with two predominating in New York and three in London: 12% of New Yorkers versus 8% of Londoners do not get out as often as they need to; 20% and 37% respectively have had less than three personal chats during the previous week (reflecting the infrequency of telephones in London). Although slightly more New Yorkers than Londoners (46% and 39% respectively) are club members, fewer New Yorkers than Londoners (21% versus 26%) have attended a club meeting in the past month. However, New Yorkers are more likely than Londoners to engage in religious activities: 53% and 39% respectively are active members of a religious congregation; and 35% and 13% respectively regularly attend church services.

It appears that differences between New York and London are not in the realm of a general tendency for subjects in one or other city to be non-participants, but rather the differences are with respect to non-participation in specific activitites.

Current Isolation. The mean scores on this scale are much the same in the two cities (5.05 in New York and 5.19 in London). Although scores of 7 or more are twice as frequent in New York as in London (33.3% vs. 17.9%), the Kolmogorov-Smirnov test shows no significant differences between the distribution of scores in the two cities (Table 3-18).

The list of items in this scale (see Table 3-19), all of which deal with numbers of social contacts during the past month, shows that New York elderly have seen more relatives and friends in the past month and belong to more clubs, while the London elderly have a greater number of contacts with siblings. Their contacts with children are nearly equal.

Total Environmental Disadvantage. The mean score on the rational scale of environmental disadvantage in New York (2.61) is close to that in London (2.54) but the Kolmogorov-Smirnov test is significant at the .01 level of confidence suggesting that the distributions of scores in the two cities are different from each other. Cumulative scores on this scale show that people in New York have a greater proportion of high scores (reflecting disadvantage) than the people in London (Table 3-20). Over 15 percent of the New York elderly and 10.6% of the London elderly score 6 or more on this scale. There are also more subjects with low scores in New York than in London (30.0% vs. 15.2% with scores of 0). Thus both high and low scorers (the extremes) predominate in New York.

The items in this scale include lack of telephone access, lack of privacy, inadequate heat, poor access to the residence, inadequate facilities, crime and a deteriorating neighborhood (Table 3-21). For 10 of the 39 items measuring environmental disadvantage the proportion of positive responders does not exceed 2% in both cities. Of the remaining 29 items, 20 predominate in New York, 7 in London, and 2 are equal in proportion of positive responders in the two cities. In all but 7 cases of predominance in one or other city, the cross-national discrepancy is 50% or more of the base figure. The environmental disadvantages predominating in New York have to do mainly with access to the residence, inadequate heat, and experience of crime, while those predominating in London are concerned mainly with lack of facilities (e.g., telephone, refrigerator, private and indoor toilet, and bathroom in apartment).

Certain of the items in this scale demonstrate particularly striking cross-national differences: no telephone in the apartment (6% vs. 41% in New York and London respectively); no toilet in the apartment (0% vs. 8%); no bathroom in the apartment (0% vs. 10%); no refrigerator (1% vs. 11%); crime involving property in past year (8% vs. 4%); not enough heat in the apartment (13% vs. 4%); and access to home a problem (12% vs. 4%).

It cannot be said that the environment of the elderly is consistently harsher in one city than in the other, but in some aspects there are striking cross-national differences, some in favor of one city and some in favor of the other.

Financial Disadvantage. The mean score on the rational scale of financial disadvantage is higher in London (1.04) than in New York (.75), and the Kolmogorov-Smirnov test is significant at the .01 level of confidence. However, this scale is composed of only 5 items so that the total scores or cumulative scores obscure rather than simplify the information available from scrutiny of the individual items; therefore the cumulative scores will not be further discussed (Table 3-22). Of the 5 items in the scale, one (income below median) is not suitable for cross-national comparison, and 2 have a frequency of positive responses equal to 2% or less in both cities (Table 3-23). The other two items deal with the subject's and examiner's evaluation that financial problems exist for the subject. This evaluation indicates that such problems exist about three times as often in New York as in London (19% for both items in New York vs. 7% and 5% for the two items in London).

Subscales: The subscales are labelled arthritis, neurological impairment, heart disease, early warning signs of cancer (cancer alert), and crime. The important cross-national differences emerging in these areas have already been mentioned when items in the subscales were reviewed during discussion of the major scales of which the subscales are part (see Table 3-5).

B-2. Comparison of the Scores on the Rational Scales by Subsample

The results of the cross-national comparisons based on the whole samples in New York and London can be checked against the corresponding findings from cross-national comparisons of the random subsamples (which is a strength of the study design). The standard error of the differences of two means is calculated by reference to the distributions of scores on subsamples. The standard error is a more accurate gauge of the importance of any cross-national differences than are statistical tests of significance. We will, however, restrict this more detailed analysis to two rational scale scores of central interest in this monograph, namely depression and dementia. The corresponding data on the other rational scales can be obtained from the authors (99).

The means of the total scores for dementia for London and New York are .7 for London, 1.2 for New York, a difference of .5, which is 2-1/2 times the standard error .19 of the difference (Table 3-24).

Of louder eloquence than the standard error of the difference is the fact that the subsample of highest dementia for London barely touches the lowest subsample for New York (see Table 3-25). If complete censuses of New York and London would show a very small difference, such as .1 or .2, the chance that the subsamples would barely overlap is miniscule.

The rational scores for depression show no difference by subsample. Table 3-26 exhibits the similarities. For depression, the cross-national difference in mean scores is less than the standard error and there is cross-national overlap between the distributions of mean scores on the subsamples.

C.   Comparison of the Distribution of Scores on the Homogeneous Scales of Health and Social Problems

As previously explained, analyses based on the homogeneous scales (17, 24) serve as a useful way of confirming, refuting or adding to the corresponding analyses with the rational scales. The homogeneous scales are composed of items that are highly intercorrelated and thus amenable to succinct conceptual description. The items in the homogeneous scales overlap with those in the rational scales but are in the majority distinct.

Thirty-one homogeneous scales are shown in Table 3-27. Eight of the scales show substantial cross-national differences in their mean scores: (1) organic brain syndrome, (2) respiratory symptoms, (3) leg swelling, (4) hearing disorders, (5) financial hardship, (6) fear of crime, (7) social isolation problems, and (8) family contact problems. The Kolmogorov-Smirnov test indicates significant cross-national differences in the distributions of scores on all of these scales. The homogeneous scale of organic brain syndrome corresponds to the rational scale of dementia and supports the findings on the latter scale to the effect that in this domain there are higher scores in New York than in London. The homogeneous scale of respiratory symptoms shows a higher score in London than in New York, thus confirming the inference made on the basis of the component items in the rational scale of physical illness. The homogeneous scale of hearing disorders shows a higher mean score in London than in New York consistent with the related items frequencies in the rational scale of perceptual impairment. The homogeneous scale score of fear of crime is higher in New York than in London as are the item scores on crime from the rational scale of environmental disadvantage and the rational subscale of crime.

The homogeneous scale of social isolation problems shows a higher mean score in London than in New York; cross-national differences for the homogeneous scale of family contact problems are in the same direction. The rational scale of isolation did not show a significant difference between the two cities but also showed more isolation in London than in New York. Moreover, there are several homogeneous scales measuring different aspects of isolation but only a single rational scale in this area.

The homogeneous scale of leg swelling, with a higher mean score in London than in New York, underlines the point made in the analysis of the rational scale of physical illness that differences between the two cities do emerge for special physical syndromes rather than for overall levels of illness.

Thus it appears, at this level of analysis, there are no important conflicts between the results obtained on the rational and the homogeneous scales.

Although frequencies of individual rational scale items were discussed, the frequencies of responses to the individual component items of the homogeneous scales will not be further discussed because the internal consistency of the homogeneous scales is so high as to make it uninformative to analyze items separately from their contribution to the general construct of the scale.

D.   Intercorrelations among Rational Scales and with Demographic Variables

In our discussion of rational scales so far we have analyzed each scale separately disregarding their interdependence, if any. In this section, we examine the intercorrelations among the major rational scales in order to determine (1) which interactions must be controlled in further analysis of a particular scale and (2) which associations warrant further analysis. We cannot from these data determine the direction of a possible cause-effect relationship or whether a third causal factor underlies a given association between a pair of scales; however, we will advance some speculations on likely causal links.

Table 3-28, giving the intercorrelations among scales, is so arranged that the top member of every pair of rows gives the data for New York and the bottom member the data for London. Significance levels are also given though we emphasize that it is the size and implications of a correlation that gives it importance rather than its being significantly different from zero.

The highest correlation is in New York between immobility and inadequate activity (.65) and the next highest correlation is for the same two scales in London (.56). This correlation is not surprising since the loss of physical abilites which are measured by the scale of immobility might be expected to limit the performance of tasks and participation in activities that are measured by the scale of inadequate activities. This finding, taken in conjunction with the lower correlations of inadequate activities with physical illness (New York .39, London .24) and with dementia (New York .28, London .25), suggest that it is immobility rather than physical illness or mental inability which is the dominant direct cause of inadequate activity in both cities.

The correlation between physical illness and immobility is strikingly high in New York (.52) but lower in London (.33); the latter correlation being about the same as the correlation between dementia and immobility in either city (New York .33 and London .30). Both physical illness and dementia appear to be major causes of immobility in the two cities.

Physical illness, immobility and inadequate activities are, as we have seen, highly related to each other. These dimensions form a cluster which reflects frailty in an elderly person. We have also pointed out that dementia attaches to this frailty cluster through its association with immobility and inadequate activities. All of these associations have face validity. However, a fifth scale, that of depression, also fits into this cluster unexpectedly firmly in New York and, to a lesser extent, in London. The place of depression in the frailty cluster raises several pertinent questions for further examination, namely, (1) what aspects of frailty are related to depression; (2) does depression cause illness, immobility and inactivity or simply arise from those states, and (3) why are the relationships with depression, especially for immobility and inactivity, higher in New York than in London? A path analysis of homogeneous scales (24), suggests that while disability causes depression, the converse is not true.

The scale of perceptual impairment also adheres to the frailty cluster described above but the strength of the associations is generally weaker than those discussed above. The relationship between depression and perceptual impairment (New York .17 and London .13) is worth noting.

The low relationship between the symptoms of depression and those of dementia suggests that these mental problems are relatively independent of each other; though the strength of the correlation differs between New York (.14) and London (-.01).

There is an inverse relationship between several of the rational scales and isolation. In addition, a strong association (shown in Table 3-28) exists in New York with inadequate activities (.34) and a weaker corresponding association in London (.14). These findings raise a question about whether isolates are better supplied with social services in London than in New York.

The lack of substantial correlation between isolation and depression in either city (.04 in New York and .01 in London) is surprising. It is plausible that isolation is a depressing situation but the empirical evidence contradicts this plausible assumption at least for the measure of isolation used here.

The intercorrelations of the rational scales with demographic variables are shown in Tables 3-29, 3-30 and 3-31.

Every one of the rational scales shows an important association with one or more demographic variables indicating the necessity of controlling (i.e., partialling out) the effects of these demographic variables when making cross-national comparisons of scores on the rational scales.

Correlations of particular interest are as follows (parentheses indicate correlations in New York and London in that order):

(1)   For age, with dementia (.25 and .29); with immobility (.31 and .37); with perceptual impairment (.22 and .28); and with inadequate activity (.23 and .19). In addition, the correlation of age with isolation is higher in London (.18) than in New York (.04), i.e., increasing age in London is associated with increasing isolation more so than in New York.

(2)   For sex, with dementia (.11 and .14); and depression (.12 and .12). The correlation of sex with financial disadvantage is much higher in New York (.17) than in London (.01).

(3)   For monthly income, there is, as expected, an inverse correlation with financial disadvantage in both cities (-.26 and -.17, respectively), since low income was scored as an item in Financial Disadvantage.

(4)   For education and occupation (Table 3-30), there are negative correlations with dementia in both cities (-.19/-.19 in New York; -.14/-.12 in London); with inadequate activities (-.10/-.01 and -.16/-.14 respectively); with financial disadvantage in New York but not in London (-.17/-.14 and -.04/-.01) and with environmental disadvantage (-.09/-.14 and -.04/-.12). Other correlations with the rational scales are less striking.

(5)   For race (Table 3-31), there are substantial differences in mean scores of dementia in New York (non-whites higher than whites) but not in London; in financial disadvantage in New York (non-whites higher than whites) but again not in London; and in isolation for New York

only (non-whites more isolated than whites). In London, the non-white group is, however, of negligible size (only 7 out of 396 subjects).

(6)   For marital status (Table 3-31), the unmarried have higher scores than the married on dementia (1.41 vs. 1.00 respectively in New York, and .88 vs. .44 in London); on immobility (3.12 vs. 2.09, and 3.43 vs. 1.94); on perceptual impairment, mainly in London (2.55 vs. 1.78); on financial disadvantage, only in New York (.99 vs. .48), and on environmental disadvantage (2.89 vs. 2.35, and 2.83 vs. 2.25).

(7)   Those living alone are in both cities more likely to be physically ill, immobile and perceptually impaired (though these relationships are statistically significant only in London); more likely to be environmentally disadvantaged; but less likely to have inadequate activities.

In summary, the correlations of rational scales and demographic variables show that with advancing age dementia, disability and social restrictions increase in both cities; that rates of mental disorder differ between the sexes; that race is related to frequency of dementia in New York, but in London the population is practically homogeneous with respect to race; that the higher educational and/or occupational ranks have lower dementia scores and less inadequate activities; that the unmarried group relative to the married are disadvantaged mentally, physically and socially in both cities; and that those living alone are more likely to be physically deteriorated than the remainder of the elderly population. These relationships will be taken into account in the more substantive analyses and discussions that follow in subsequent sections of this book. However, the impression gained from these data is that the associations of health and social problems is by and large the same in the two cities; cross-national similarities are the rule and differences the exception.

3.   THE PREVALENCE OF THE CATEGORIES OF DEPRESSION AND OF DEMENTIA

In the preceding sections we have examined cross-national discrepancies in rational and homogeneous scale scores and in the frequency of responses on individual items in the CARE. We now consider the cross-national comparison of categories of psychiatric problems within the areas of depression and dementia.

Experience with Face-to-Face Diagnosis. A face-to-face "provisional" psychiatric diagnosis was made in those cases where the project interviewer was a psychiatrist, which was in all cases in London and a random half of the cases in New York. Diagnosis was made according to the descriptions of the International Classification of Diseases (ICD), 9th Edition, and the accompanying glossary of terms (100). The reliability of this diagnostic system with geriatric patients has been established for the project psychiatrists in a prior study (40), which, however, was based on inpatients. The reliability for diagnosis on community subjects was attempted in a formal study but, as it transpired, the low prevalence rates of severe psychiatric conditions in the community did not allow an adequate representation of these conditions in the sample examined during the systematic reliability study. Furthermore, the psychiatrists found difficulty in applying the ICD criteria to community subjects, for reasons that will be detailed later. Thus a review process was developed to submit all cases to classification by explicit and specific criteria designed especially to diagnose depression or dementia in the community elderly. This process allowed all cases to be diagnosed including not only those interviewed by psychiatrists but also those interviewed by the social scientists and psychologists on the project team. It also allowed a consensus to be reached by project psychiatrists in both cities with respect to psychiatric diagnoses on both New York and London samples.

In the discussion that follows the label "depression," if unqualified, is an umbrella term for all types of depression: normal reactions to life's vicissitudes, life dissatisfaction, demoralization syndromes, grief reactions as well as neurotic and psychotic depressions, major and minor affective disorders, manic-depressive disorders, involutional melancholia, endogenous depression, reactive psychotic depression, and unipolar and bipolar depressions. All these conditions have in common a tendency to depressed mood, excessive worry, apathy, tension, and pessimism. Various symptoms, the course of the illness and etiological associations allow subclassification of the depressive sub-types. The label "clinical depression" refers to those depressions which are sufficiently persistent, disruptive or severe to warrant skilled evaluation and treatment by a health care professional. The label later introduced of "pervasive depression" is very similar to clinical depression but has specific criteria which warrants a distinctive label.

Similarly, the label "dementia," if unqualified, is a shorthand synonym for organic brain syndrome, characterized mainly by disorientation and memory impairment. Various symptoms, the course of the illness and its etiological associations allow organic brain syndrome to be subclassified into acute (confusional states) and chronic types, and the latter into benign and malignant or progressive types. The progressive dementias can be further classified into the secondary and primary kinds. The most common subtypes of the primary progressive dementias are senile dementia (often called the Alzheimer type) and arteriosclerotic or multi-infarct dementia. The label "clinical dementia" refers to the progressive dementias. The label later described of pervasive dementia is very similar to clinical dementia but has specific criteria which warrant a distinctive label.

        Some   Difficulties   in   Making   Diagnoses   in   the Community. An important issue in judging the relative merits of diagnostic systems for use in the community is the extent to which they are helpful in making decisions about 'caseness.' The determination of who is a case is usually based on clinical judgement. Where a diagnosis of psychiatric disorder has been made by a psychiatrist it is implicit that that person is a case in the view of that psychiatrist. However, it became apparent in the course of this community study that the psychiatrists at face-to-face interviews were proceeding as if the placement of a person in a category of psychiatric disorder was a separate process and not an inherent part of judging whether that person was a case. For example there was a frequent use of qualifiers of caseness attached to the diagnosis such as the terms early, slight, or possible (depression or dementia). These qualifiers were disproportionately used by some of the project psychiatrists suggesting, as one might expect, that they are not reliable terms. Moreover, these qualifiers, generally indicating uncertainty about caseness, were much more evident than indications of uncertainty about the distinction between depression and dementia (as when paired as preferred and alternative diagnoses). Perhaps it is not surprising that psychiatrists find differential diagnosis easier than case determination since their experience is primarily with clinic populations where it is taken for granted that someone who attends as a patient is a case and the diagnostic task is simply to differentially assign the patient to a category of diagnosis.

        Unfortunately, the diagnostic manuals currently available do not provide explicit criteria for case determination even where these are provided for differential diagnosis. Nor can a present or past history of receiving psychiatric treatment be a satisfactory epidemiological criterion of being a case. Putting aside the possibility that some patients attending psychiatric clinics are not in fact cases (by plausible criteria independent of the fact of attendance), it is likely that many persons not attending psychiatric clinics are cases by such plausible criteria. This likelihood will vary with the prediliction of a particular population for seeking psychiatric treatment and with the availability of such services. Indeed an important research question might be whether cases are more likely to receive psychiatric treatment in one community setting rather than another. Thus, cross-national or other group comparisons would be confounded by adopting as a criterion for case definition the fact of being or having been, for example, an attender at a psychiatric clinic or an inpatient in a psychiatric ward.

A major advantage of the new community diagnostic system (i.e., pervasive depression and dementia) is the attention given to case determination.

The Review Process. It will be recalled, that all subjects were rated on discrete items of psychopathology whose reliability was established between project interviewers within and across the disciplines of psychiatry, social science, and psychology. In addition, global ratings of degree of psychiatric impairment were made at interview (14). The discrete items were scored on rational scales of depression and dementia and according to latent class analysis of these two parameters (16). Thus there were three non-diagnostic sources of information indicating the likelihood of a person being depressed or demented: the rational score, latent class and global impairment. These three sources of information were used to screen all subjects to identify those requiring intensive review.

A score of 6 or more on the rational scales of either depression or dementia was selected as a cutting point for including subjects for further review, on the grounds that few face-to-face diagnoses of depression or dementia were made by project psychiatrists on subjects whose scores did not reach these cutting points.

For the global rating of impairment a cutting score of 4 or more was established on similar grounds to those described in the preceding paragraph and also because the anchoring definition for this level of score calls for moderate or severe symptoms (marked anxiety, deep depression, marked memory impairment, etc.).

Therefore all subjects were included for further review who scored six or more on the rational scale; or who scored four or more on the global rating of psychiatric impairment; as a further safeguard against missing possible cases all subjects were included for review who had a probability greater than .90 of fitting the latent classes of dementia or depression. The numbers of subjects produced for review in this fashion were as follows: rational scales, 115 New York respondents (26%) and 87 London respondents (22%); latent class assignment, 83 New Yorkers (19%) and 86 Londoners (22%); and global scales of impairment, 124 New Yorkers (28%) and 53 Londoners (13%). Since these were overlapping numbers the totals of subjects for review, 172 (39%) in New York and 142 (36%) in London were less than an additive score of the subjects produced by each of the three components of the screen (see Table 3-32). The subjects selected for the review process were therefore based on a screening process which employed data of known and good reliability.

The extent to which possible cases of dementia or depression slipped through this screen will be examined but requires first a description of the manner in which specific criteria were applied to produce the final diagnosis.

The Application of the New Diagnostic Criteria. The criteria used in final diagnosis have been published elsewhere (10, 14). These criteria (Appendices I and II) were developed especially for application to the kind of information that can be obtained by use of the CARE, and with awareness of the difficulties of diagnosis in the elderly community subject. The main features of this set of criteria are as follows: (1) the components of the criteria are defined and in most instances the definition is based on a specific CARE item; (2) the components of the criteria can be synthesized into a diagnosis by following the guidelines; (3) the criteria relate both to the pattern of symptoms and to their severity so that both these parameters (i.e., pattern and severity) can be used to describe cases or follow progress; (4) non-clinical states of depression or dementia (i.e., distress or impairment which do not appear to warrant clinical attention), as well as clinical states, are classified; (5) symptom patterns, social adjustment, positive mental health, stress, associated conditions and course of illness are all taken into account in the diagnostic criteria; (6) the criteria provide for the distinction between symptoms which are the product of psychiatric disturbance and those due to physical disease (a difficult but important distinction in the case of symptoms such as sleep disturbance or autonomic symptoms); (7) the distinction between the memory changes of dementia, depression and normal aging is aided by the criteria; and (8) subtypes of clinical depression or dementia are identified.

The reliability of applying these new criteria was tested in the following manner. One hundred and twenty-four personal time dependent cases* from the New York sample were chosen for review and their narrative summaries were censored

---

*This subsample, composed of personal time dependent subjects (as defined in a later section), might be expected to include a higher proportion of dementias than would be found in the full cross-section sample, which also helped to facilitate carrying out this diagnostic exercise.

to remove references to diagnosis. The narrative summaries, as mentioned in the section on Methods, had been written after each interview according to systematic guidelines, namely (1) all important mental, physical and social symptoms elicited by the CARE interview should be recorded as directly as possible (i.e., without unnecessary interpretation) so that another rater could independently judge their implications; (2) the chronology of the symptoms, previous health problems, treatment received and its effects, and unfulfilled treatment needs should be described; and, (3) evidence of positive assets (health or social) should be listed as defined in the global ratings.

The non-psychiatrists, who were specially trained research assistants, independently applied the diagnostic criteria of pervasive depression or dementia to the summaries. The raters also reviewed the profile of rational scale scores when in doubt. A satisfactory level of reliability was obtained for both depression and dementia. There is a 93% agreement, with a Kappa of .73 on Pervasive Dementia (Table 3-33) and a 90% agreement, with a Kappa of .75 on Pervasive Depression (Table 3-34). The statistic Kappa is a measure of the extent of agreement between raters, corrected for the amount of agreement which might be expected by chance alone. It varies from 0 (no more agreement than would be expected by chance) to 1 (complete agreement).

The screened cases (172 in New York and 142 in London) were all reviewed by one project psychiatrist who applied the specific criteria to the systematic narrative summaries (censored to remove reference to diagnostic judgements), and the profiles of rational scores covering psychiatric, medical and social syndromes. This application of the criteria for diagnosis to the cases selected for review produced the distributions shown in Table 3-36. The term "pervasive depression," as previously described, indicates cases of depression that meet the specific criteria; these cases are at a clinical level of severity, i.e., assumed to warrant the attention of a health care professional skilled in the treatment of psychiatric disturbance. Similarly, "pervasive dementia" refers to cases of dementia that are expected to generally follow a progressively disabling course. More detailed definitions of these terms are given in the criteria.

The CARE interview is aimed at identifying symptoms which are present at, or during the month prior to, interview (though historical information is included in the process of classification). In practice, this emphasis on current symptomatology means that the rates reported are those of point prevalence. These rates are shown in Table 3-35.

The prevalence rates of pervasive depression show a surprising similarity between New York (13.0%) and London (12.4%). In contrast, the prevalence of pervasive dementia in New York is over twice that in London (4.9 and 2.3 percent respectively). These results are consistent with the data reported in a previous section on the distribution of scores on the rational scales of depression and dementia.

False Negatives. In order to detect the presence of false negatives in diagnosis arising from possible insensitivity of the screening criteria (i.e., rational scores, latent classes, and global impairment ratings) the following procedure was carried out: the data on those subjects in which the interviewer was a psychiatrist (all in London and half in New York) were scrutinized to identify subjects receiving a face-to-face (provisional) diagnosis of any psychiatric disorder but who had not met the screening criteria. Diagnoses that were qualified by such terms as mild, early, doubtful or possible were disregarded. Only unqualified diagnoses or those described as moderate, severe, definite or clinical were accepted. These subjects (provisional diagnosis positive but screen negative) were mixed in with the subjects who were positive on the screening criteria and all were subjected to the final diagnostic review process as previously described. False negatives were defined as those subjects who received a diagnosis of pervasive depression or pervasive dementia but did not meet the screening criteria. The number of cases that received a diagnosis of pervasive depression or pervasive dementia was 80 in New York and 58 in London. Every one of these cases met the screening criteria in New York; and in London, all but two. Thus there were no false negatives in New York; and in London, only two, both of which received a diagnosis of pervasive depression. These results show that the results of the cross-national comparison of rates of depression and dementia are not likely to have been influenced by insensitivity on the part of the screening stage of the diagnostic review process.

We are assuming that there were no subjects who would have received a diagnosis of depression or dementia among those who were negative on the screen and also were judged at face-to-face interview not to warrant a provisional diagnosis of a psychiatric disorder. This assumption is supported by evidence that the screen was, as intended, over-inclusive. As previously stated, the screen identified 172 possible cases in New York and 142 in London for review, but of these possible cases only 80 in New York and 58 in London were given a diagnosis of pervasive depression or pervasive dementia.

Case Definition. Because this study has both health service and etiological interests, we wish to identify two different though overlapping types of cases in the community:

(1) those whose psychiatric symptoms were enough to warrant intervention by a health care professional (not necessarily a psychiatrist), and (2) those whose symptoms are characteristic of a specific psychiatric disorder.

For the first type of case definition mentioned above (i.e., warranting professional intervention), we have distinguished between symptoms which do not dominate the person's life (i.e., are limited) and those which do (i.e., are pervasive).

The second type (specific psychiatric disorder) is largely a subset of the first type (warranting professional intervention). The hallmarks of a specific disorder are found in the symptom patterns (e.g., the conjunction of mood disturbance with certain somatic symptoms), the relationship to a stressful event (e.g., bereavement or head injury), the association with other disorders (e.g., the association with mania in the case of depression or with Parkinson's disease in the case of dementia), the premorbid adjustment and the development and course of the condition. These features being partly historical and partly inferential are generally not as reliably assessed as the more current and observable features listed in the first type of case definition, or require more extensive investigation and observation than is usually available in an epidemiological study. Hence we have preferred for our purposes to use the diagnoses of pervasive depression or dementia. However, the sequential sorting of subjects with the pervasive diagnoses in the process of arriving at specific psychiatric disorder is displayed in Figures 3-1 and 3-2. For example, the criteria for the diagnosis of manic-depressive-depressive disorder (a subtype of pervasive depression), require the presence of pervasive depression, somatic (vegetative) symptoms, an associated level of stress not sufficient to explain the intensity of the symptoms, and a history of episodic illness; each step in the application of these criteria is displayed separately. The most reliable step is put first and the most complex and inferential last.

Rates of Depression and Dementia by Various Criteria. The analysis of prevalence rates has so far been concentrated on the categories in which we have the greatest confidence, namely, pervasive depression and pervasive dementia. However, we need to know to what extent the cross-national differences are restricted to the particular criteria applied. If a similar cross-national trend is shown for a domain of psychopathology (e.g., morbid depression) no matter what the criteria for classification then the results will be mutually reinforcing. Table 3-36 shows the cross-national comparison of prevalence rates of classes of depression and dementia by various criteria and demonstrates that the ratio of the rates in New York compared to those in

London follow the same trend for almost all of the criteria applied; namely the relative rates for depression are much the same in the two cities while the relative rates for dementia are more than twice as high in New York as in London. The absolute rates of course differ depending on the criteria applied.

The exception is that, contrary to the cross-national trend for depression, manic-depressive-depressive disorders are twice as common in New York as in London.   However, reference to the diagrams of sequential diagnosis (Figures 3-1 and 3-2) will show that this cross-national difference emerged only when the criterion relating to the episodic nature of the disorder was taken into account. This historical information is not sufficiently reliable to warrant any inferences to be drawn about this cross-national difference; especially in the absence of the kind of reinforcing evidence that occurs with dementia (i.e., trends shown by other criteria in the same domain).

A.   An Analysis of the Excess Rates of Dementia in New York Compared with London

In the previous sections we presented data which suggested that there are higher rates of dementia in New York than in London. We referred to a range of data: the distribution of scores on the rational scale of dementia (essentially the symptoms of organic brain syndrome), the latent class of dementia (a statistical method of clustering persons on the basis of their symptoms), and the diagnosis of the dementing conditions by use of explicit and reliable criteria.   Whichever of the indicators of dementia are invoked, the rates are found to be about two times higher in New York than in London.   In this section we look for straightforward explanations of these findings by examination of related data.

The indicators of dementia we have used are highly related to each other. For example, 15 out of the 22 cases diagnosed as pervasive dementia in New York had scores of 6 or more on the rational scale of dementia; in London 8 out of 9. Conversely, 15 out of the 26 persons in New York with scores of 6 or more on the rational scale of dementia were diagnosed as pervasive dementia; in London 8 out of 10. Therefore, for convenience, we will focus our explanatory analyses on only one indicator; we have chosen the rational scale of dementia. The use of a scale rather than a diagnostic category for the analyses will facilitate the calculations required because it provides a continuous score as well as a category that can be formed by reference to a cut-off score.   Corresponding comparisons involving other indicators of dementia are described elsewhere (14).

Figure 3-1. Sequential Classification of Dementia in New York
and London (definitions of all terms in the
Appendix)

Dementia in New York:

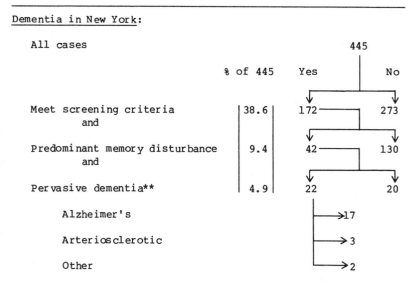

All cases   445

                          % of 445   Yes   No

Meet screening criteria   38.6   172   273
        and

Predominant memory disturbance 9.4   42   130
        and

Pervasive dementia**   4.9   22   20

        Alzheimer's   →17

        Arteriosclerotic   → 3

        Other   → 2

Dementia in London:

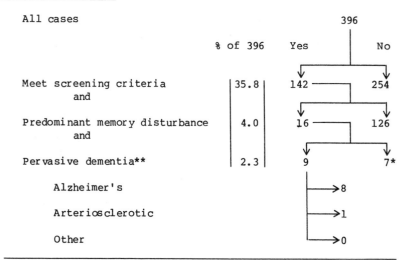

All cases   396

                          % of 396   Yes   No

Meet screening criteria   35.8   142   254
        and

Predominant memory disturbance 4.0   16   126
        and

Pervasive dementia**   2.3   9   7*

        Alzheimer's   → 8

        Arteriosclerotic   → 1

        Other   → 0

*One case of acute confusional state.
**Domain of chronic organic brain syndrome.

As a first step in the analytic strategy the demographic and rational scales' associations with dementia are explored. The demographic variables with correlations of .10 or higher with scores on the rational scale of dementia are age, race, sex, educational level, professional occupation, and marital status (see Table 3-37).

Since the listed demographic variables correlate with dementia it is necessary to control for their possible effect on relative rates of dementia in the two cities. It is difficult to control this many variables at the same time even with sample sizes of several hundred persons and a step-wise multiple regression analysis was carried out to select the variables accounting for most of the variance in the scores of dementia. Age was found to account for about 8% of the variance in both New York and London with only sex adding a significant amount to this figure and the other variables even less.

The demographic group containing most of the persons who score 6 or more on the rational scale of dementia in New York can be characterized as very old, women who are either non-white or are foreign born and in the lower SES groups. A path analysis (24) suggests that age is the major determinant of the relationship between dementia and this multidimensional demographic group. Thus an age control introduced into the cross-national comparison is a crucial control over demographic effects.

Age and Sex. The cross-national comparison of rates of dementia was repeated controlling for age and sex; the results are shown in Table 3-38. The excess of dementia in New York compared to London remains after adjusting the figures within each sex group to discount the effects of age on cross-national differences in rates of dementia.

Education. In an earlier section we discussed the cross-national differences on each item of the dementia scale and suggested that the items expected to be least affected by educational level contributed most to the excess of high dementia scores in New York compared with London. Furthermore, a regression analysis suggested that controlling for age and sex would reduce (although not eliminate) any important variance in the dementia rates of these samples due to other demographic variables such as educational level. Nevertheless, the influence of education on the cross-national comparison is sufficiently interesting to warrant further examination.

We find that the New York elderly are less educated: only 57% have an eighth grade or higher level of education compared with 88% of the London elderly. Some investigators (101, 102) have attempted to control the effects of education

Figure 3-2. Sequential Classification of Depression in New York and London (definitions of all terms in the Appendix)

Depression in New York:

	% of 445	Yes	No
All cases		445	
Meet screening criteria and	38.6	172	273
Predominantly depressed and	21.6	96	76
Pervasively depressed and	13.0	58	39
Vegetative symptoms and	6.1	24	34
Stress not overwhelming and	4.3	17	7
Episodic history*	2.8	11	6

Depression in London:

	% of 396	Yes	No
All cases		396	
Meet screening criteria and	35.8	142	254
Predominantly depressed and	19.9	78	64
Pervasively depressed and	12.4	49	27
Vegetative symptoms and	5.6	22	29
Stress not overwhelming and	4.0	15	6
Episodic history*	1.3	5	11

*Domain of major affective disorder or manic-depressive-depressive disorder or endogenous depression.

on scores of dementia by discounting one point (i.e., one error) for a group with poor education (or discounting two points if educational groups are widely separated). Table 3-39 shows the effects of this procedure. The criterion score of 6 or more errors on the rational scale of dementia is obtained by more New Yorkers than Londoners both with respect to unadjusted scores and also where one error is discounted from all New York scores; and even where two errors are so discounted.

Race and Nativity. It is probable that any effect of race and nativity on cross-national differences in rates of dementia would be accounted for by differences in education, age and sex (which have already been examined). Furthermore, the uniformity of the cross-national trends across almost all items in the dementia scale (and across the different indicators of dementia, including diagnosis) do not suggest that cultural bias with respect to the indicators of dementia are important determinants of these findings on dementia. However, the proportions of the New York and London samples who are racially white or native born are so different that further documentation of the relationship between these variables and rates of dementia in the two cities is required.

Non-white elderly persons constitute 15% of the sample in New York but only 1% of the sample in London. Removing these groups (which are too small for comparisons in their own right) from their respective samples allows a comparison of the remainder, all of whom are white. Among the latter group, the prevalence rate of persons scoring 6 or more on the rational scale of dementia is 5.2% in New York and 2.5% in London; which is in the same cross-national direction and of the same order as the overall findings on dementia.

Foreign born elderly persons constitute 61% of the New York sample but only 10% of the London sample. The latter group is too small to permit cross-national comparison of dementia rates but removing these groups allows a comparison of native born elderly persons in the two cities. The relevant rates of persons scoring 6 or more on the rational scale of dementia are 4.7% in New York and 2.5% in London; again consistent with the overall findings.

Relation Of Dementia To Other Mental And Physical Conditions. Table 3-28 shows the correlation of the rational scale of dementia with rational scales reflecting other mental and physical conditions.

The higher correlation of depression and dementia in New York (.14) than in London (-.01) might raise the question of whether some of the cases counted as dementia in the former city were in fact pseudodementias (i.e., depressions with a consequent disorder of memory). Against this possibility is evidence that depression correlates not only with dementia but with several physical conditions more highly in New York than in London; with physical illness .47 in New York and .37 in London, with immobility .42 and .15 respectively, and with perceptual impairment .17 and .13. It seems less likely that the correlation between depression and dementia is due substantially to the presence of pseudodementia than that New Yorkers are more likely to become depressed in the presence of health or mental problems than Londoners. Supporting this contention is that the findings on the relative rates of dementia in the two cities as measured by scores of 6 or more on the rational scales were supported by the findings based on diagnosis. In the latter every effort was made to exclude pseudodementia from the category of pervasive dementia by the use of specific criteria to identify memory disturbance characteristic of depression and by giving due weight to the presence of affective symptoms even where cognitive impairment co-existed { evidence for this is reported in detail elsewhere (15)}. Finally, it should be noted that since the number of caes scoring high on dementia is lower in London than in New York, the correlations are less likely to reach significance in London.

The higher correlation in New York than in London of dementia with physical illness could indicate either (1) that the physical state of these cases contributes more in New York than in London to the expression of dementia symptoms or (2) that there is corresponding cross-national difference in the maintenance of health in dementia cases or (3) that the most severely ill cases of dementia in London have died or been institutionalized. Of these possibilities, the last seems to be consistent with the finding that there are relatively more persons with very high scores of dementia in New York than in London.

The correlation of perceptual impairment and dementia in New York but not in London is surprising because as previously discussed there are higher rates of deafness in London compared with New York and no cross-national differences in visual difficulty. It is possible that deafness imposes a greater disadvantage on New Yorkers than Londoners in the domain of cognitive performance.

There is a higher correlation in London (.14) than in New York (.07) between neurological disorder (presumably stroke for the most part) and dementia but this is not supported by the diagnostic results which suggest that similar proportions of dementias in the two cities are due to cerebral arteriosclerosis or multi-infarcts.

All in all, there is no obvious explanation in these data for the excess dementia in New York; but perhaps some

supportive evidence that there are not only more cases of
dementia in New York than in London but they are probably more
severe as well.

B.   The Correlations of Depression and Age in New York and
      London

     In earlier sections we indicated that similarities
between the two cities in rates of depression overshadowed
any differences that also emerged in this domain.   Most
striking of all was that the prevalence rate of pervasive
depression   (identifying   depressions   which   warranted
professional intervention) was practically the same in the
two cities.

     A further question is whether the correlates of
depression are also similar in each city. In this section we
will have a closer look at the association between depression
and chronological age in each city.

     For most of the analyses that follow we will use the
rational scale of depression rather than the latent class or
diagnosis of depression. The use of the rational scale will
facilitate analysis because it provides a continuous score as
well as a category that can be formed by reference to a
cut-off score.   A cut-off depression score of 6 or more
defines a category that correlates highly with the latent
class and diagnosis of depression. The age patterns of other
indicators of depression are discussed elsewhere (10).

     Figures 3-3 and 3-4 show the proportion of each age
group obtaining a score of 6 or more on the rational scale of
depression. Any age group containing less than 30 subjects
was merged with the next younger age group (except for the
combined sexes groups where the age groups were not merged).
The combined sexes group shows a decreasing prevalence rate
of depression from the age category 65-69 to 75-79 in both
cities; the prevalence rate then rises in New York from the
age category 80-84 upwards while in London the prevalence
rate remains steady in the corresponding age span.

     The age trends for each sex separately show some
surprising cross-national similarities: in both cities males
have lower prevalence rates of depression than females prior
to age 75 with the ratio of rates in men to those in women
being in both cities about 2:3 at age 65-69 and 1:3 at age
70-74.   In both cities the rates for each sex converge at
about age 75-79. In New York the rates of depression in men
rise dramatically after age 75-79, exceeding those for women
by about twofold at age 80 and over; this projection is not
possible for men in London because of their small sample
size. In both cities the rates for women fall somewhat after
age 70-74.   Also striking is that in both cities, the

Figure 3-3. Proportion of New York Elderly with Scores
of 6 or more on the Rational Scale:
Depression by Age

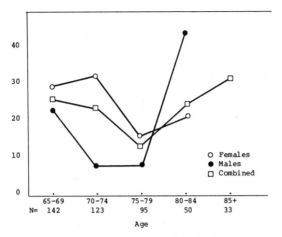

Note: The frequencies of respondents in the various age
categories were as follows: 61 males age 65-69; 48 males
age 70-74; 35 males age 75-79; 33 males over age 79; 81
females age 65-69; 75 females age 70-74; 60 females age
75-79; 50 females over age 79. For the combined sample
the frequencies are 142, 123, 95, 50, 23 and 10.

Figure 3-4. Proportion of London Elderly with Scores
of 6 or more on the Rational Scale:
Depression by Age

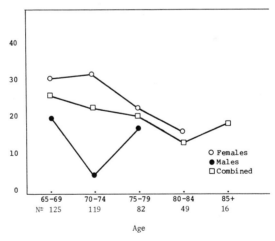

Note: The frequencies of respondents in the various age
categories were as follows: 49 males age 65-69; 41 males
age 70-74; 48 males over age 74. 76 females age 65-69;
78 females age 70-74; 48 females age 75-79; 56 females over
age 79. For the combined sample the frequencies are 125,
119, 82, 51, 13 and 6.

prevalence rate of depression in men enters a trough at age 70-74, falling from the region of 20% at age 65-69 to the region of 5-8% at age 70-74 and then rising thereafter.

Overall then, in both cities the prevalence rates of depression in females appears to subside with advancing age while for men the rates dip to a low point at age 70-74 and then rise.

The next sequence in the analysis of the relationship between depression and chronological age in the two cities is to examine the variation with age of those health and social problems that were in a previous section shown to be correlated with depression. This age variation is shown in Table 3-40. The identification of correlates of depression which also show the same age variation as depression might help to explain the latter phenomenon.

In males, the age pattern characteristic of depression (a dip in rate at 70-74, highest rates in oldest age groups) is shown by physical illness in both New York and London, and by financial dissatisfaction and immobility in New York but not in London. We now restrict ourselves to the scales consistent in males with their age pattern of depression; we find that in females, age patterns consistent with that characteristic of female depression (fairly level or, if anything, somewhat higher at 65-74 than at 75 or above) are shown by physical illness and by financial disadvantage, but not by immobility, in both New York and London. Other scales which show an age pattern consistent with that of depression in females (environmental disadvantage and isolation) do not show the characteristic age pattern of depression in males. Thus the most consistent parallel with the age variation of depression (i.e., in both sexes and both cities) is shown by the rational scale of physical illness. (Note: the male age group 80+ years in London contains only 14 subjects so that the rates in that group are interpreted with reserve.)

The most parsimonious explanation of the observed age variation in depression appears to be a causal relationship to physical illness. However, these data also suggest the possibility that factors predisposing to depression in elderly women differ from those pertaining to elderly men. It is also impossible in these data to separate the effects of age from cohort (or generational) effects as discussed more fully elsewhere (18).

A key observation based on these data is once again, that the associations of mental disorders are more similar than dissimilar in the two cities.

4. PERSONAL TIME DEPENDENCY

The chronic mental and physical infirmities that accompany old age make the elderly population vulnerable to becoming dependent on others for help in coping with the demands of their environment. The help that is needed often involves the providers of that help in a time-consuming task: their personal time is required. The state of dependency requiring time-consuming help from another person, which is the major focus of this section, will be called "personal time dependency" (PTD).

Measurement of Personal Time Dependency: Persons with (1) mental or physical disabilities that cause (2) inability to perform tasks which (3) requires someone to spend time providing services in direct contact with the dependent (4) and the withholding of the service would seriously threaten the dependent's continued existence in that setting (i.e., existence would become impossible or intolerable) were defined as personal time dependent.

Table 3-41 shows the kinds of disabilities associated with dependency and the services required to care for them. Actually, all members of society are accustomed to receive services as part of the exchanges of social life. Those services, such as general retailing, public transport, friendly relations, housing, etc., which are not usually signs of personal time dependency as defined here, have been excluded. It is possible, however, that a healthy member of the community can also receive services listed in the table, not because of disability or necessity, but because of habit or convenience. For this reason, services and disabilities have been placed in adjacent columns, since in order to define dependency, an inference must be made that people who receive services have a corresponding disability which requires the service to support them in the community.

The judgement of personal time dependency requires therefore the following sequence of decisions. First the rater determines whether the respondent receives any of the service listed in Table 3-41. Second, he notes inability to perform certain tasks as reported or revealed by observation. Third, the rater decides whether the services correspond to the inability. Fourth, other evidence is weighed as to whether the inability is due to mental or physical causes, i.e., is a disability. Finally, the rater makes a judgement, based on the severity of disability, whether if services were withdrawn then the disability would seriously threaten continued existence in that setting. If the latter judgement is affirmative, if the services and the inability match, and if evidence for a mental or physical origin is judged to be present, then and only then is it assumed that a personal time dependency exists.

One hundred and four randomly selected cases were independently reviewed by two trained but non-medical raters in order to determine the reliability of these judgements. The level of agreement between the two raters for the prevalence of personal time dependency was 90%, with a Kappa of .78 as is shown in Table 3-42.

In order to determine what kinds of disability were reflected in the judgements on the presence of personal time dependency, we reviewed the CARE schedule and listed all items which seemed relevant to the construct of personal time dependency. These items were then correlated with the dependency ratings. Twenty-nine items with Pearson correlation coefficients higher than .30 were selected to form a highly reliable scale with an internal consistency of .94 in New York and .92 in London (Cronbach's Alpha) (103). This scale correlated .83 with the judgmental ratings of dependency, giving further evidence of the reliability of the judgments. Table 3-43 shows the items and their correlation with the total score. These reflect different problems in functioning that when severe or frequent enough, result in a clinical rating of dependency. The items in this scale give a picture of the disabilities in the two cities. All ratings, unless otherwise specified, were based on the subject's status and circumstances in the past month.

Results: The proportion of the elderly that fulfills the criteria for PTD is 30% in New York and 31% in London; nearly identical. The distribution of these personal time dependents in each city were then compared with respect to a number of demographic variables. Table 3-44 summarizes the results.

We see that even though the overall dependency rate is the same in the two cities the distribution is different among the demographic groups. In London compared with New York, PTDs are a higher proportion of the following groups: never married, divorced or separated, widowed, and those living alone. These groups have in common that they have relatively weak community (i.e., informal) supports compared, for example, to the married group (where the cross-national rates of dependency are similar). It is also interesting to note the reverse trends in the two cities regarding frequency of PTDs by neighborhood type. In New York dependent subjects tend to be most concentrated in poor neighborhoods and are most highly represented among Blacks, Hispanics, and Protestants, while in London they tend to be most concentrated in good neighborhoods and are disproportionately found among Catholics.

The two dependent groups (i.e., in New York and London) do not differ much from each other with regard to their distribution among gender, or nativity groups. The relationship between age and PTD in New York and London is also similar. Table 3-45 illustrates that in both cities the PTDs increase serially as a proportion of each older age group so that there is nearly twice as high a proportion of PTDs in the age group 80 and over as below that age, but there are still almost twice as many PTDs in absolute numbers below age 80 (N = 85 New York, 82 London) as above that age (N = 46 New York, 42 London).

Table 3-46 shows the relationship between, on the one hand, the scores on the rational scales as indices of health and social problems and, on the other hand, the presence and levels of severity of PTD in the two cities. In order to add interest to this analysis, these conditions have been clustered arbitrarily into those which are possible causes of PTD; those which are possible effects; and a third group which are possible modifiers acting between disability and degree of dependence. The third group is called "possible disadvantages" in that these situations are presumed to make it more difficult to cope with PTD if it exists.

The correlations between the rational scale scores and PTD are cross-nationally similar with the exception of financial disadvantage where the correlation is significant in New York but not in London. Some conditions do have higher mean scores in one city than the other (e.g., dementia is higher in New York and perceptual impairment is higher in London), but in those instances the higher scores occur for both dependents and independents. Apparently almost all the same conditions are associated with PTD in the two cities as possible causes, effects and disadvantages.

In both cities, among the indices designated as possible causes, it is dementia and neurological disorder that are the most marked and regular associations of both the presence and severity of dependence. Arthritis and perceptual disorder, however, seem to be associated regularly with the presence but not the severity of dependence.

The presence and severity of dependence appear to be more closely associated in New York than in London with the possible effects indicated by depression and inadequate activities. This is shown more clearly for depression in Figure 3-5. The cumulative frequency of depression is cross-nationally similar for the independent elderly but cumulative frequencies shift further towards higher depressive scores for the PTDs in New York than they do in London.

The indicator of depression in Table 3-47, the diagnosis of pervasive depression, is an index of a serious level of depression of clear interest to the health service

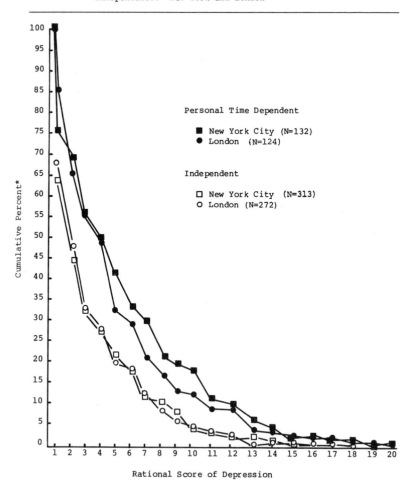

Figure 3-5. Cumulative Percent* Distribution of Rational
Scores on Depression for Dependents and
Independents: New York and London

Rational Score of Depression

*Percent with indicated score or greater.

system. Such a level of depression occurs in 16% of New York PTD's and 18% of London PTD's.

It would seem that the clinical depressions are equally high in the PTD's of New York and London but that the broader concept of depression (including demoralization)implicit in the rational scale scores of depression is more closely associated with dependency in New York than in London.

Table 3-2. Comparison of New York City Census* Demographics to New York Community Sample (in percents)

	Estimated July 1, 1976* %	New York Community Study 1975-1976 %
Proportion of elderly over age 75	35%	40%
Sex distribution		
Males	39	40
Females	61	60
Males by age		
65 - 74	65	62
75 and above	35	38
Females by age		
65 - 74	65	60
75 and above	35	40

*N.Y. State Economic Development Board, Preliminary Revised Population Projections by Age and Sex for New York, March 1976.

Table 3-1 appears on page 66.

Table 3-1.   Demographic Characteristics of New York and London
             Elderly (in percents)

Characteristic	New York (N=445)	London (N=396)
<u>Age</u>		
Mean age	74 yrs.	74 yrs.
Proportion over 75	40%	38%
Females		
65-70 yrs.	30	30
71-75 yrs.	28	30
76-80 yrs.	23	19
81+ yrs.	19	22
Males		
65-70 yrs.	35	36
71-75 yrs.	27	30
76-80 yrs.	20	25
81+ yrs.	19	10
<u>Sex</u>		
Males	40	35
Females	60	65
<u>Ethnicity/Race</u>		
White	85	99
Black	10	1
Hispanic	4	0
Other	6	0
<u>Religion</u>		
Roman Catholic	39	10
Jewish	35	3
Protestant	14	17
Church of England	4	62
Other	9	9
<u>Country of Origin</u>		
Native	39	90
Foreign	61	10
<u>Occupation</u> (Most of Life)		
White Collar	30	30
Blue Collar	42	37
Unskilled, Service	11	23
Housewife	17	10
<u>Marital Status</u>		
Now Married	46	47
Widowed	41	39
Divorced/Separated	5	3
Never Married	7	11

Note: In some cases %'s total slightly less or slightly more
       than 100% due to rounding error.

Table 3-3. Comparison of Greater London Census* Demographics
to London Community Sample (in percents)

	London* 1976 %	London Community Study 1975-1976 %
Proportion of elderly over age 75	36%	38%
Sex distribution		
Males	38	35
Females	62	65
Males by age		
65 - 74	64	66
75 and above	36	34
Females by age		
65 - 74	59	59
75 and above	41	41

*1976 Annual Abstract of Greater London Statistics, Vol. II,
H.M.S.O.

Table 3-4.   Life-Style Characteristics of New York and London
             Elderly (in percents)

Characteristic	New York (N=445) %	London (N=396) %
Social Contacts		
Living alone	31	33
Not even one child living	27	25
No visitors in the past month	16	12
No confidante	12	20
Club member	46	39
Member of a congregation	53	39
Little time in recreation	10	7
Getting out		
Almost never	8	7
1-6 days a week	22	27
Each day	69	66
Crime		
Crime victim in past year	4	1
Facilities		
No phone	7	41
No refrigerator	1	10
No bathing facility	0	10
Housing		
Neighborhood deteriorating	38	34
Median years at current address	17 yrs.	15 yrs.
Median number of rooms	4	4
Dwelling self-owned	28	22
Self-contained apartment in purpose built building	62	34
Self-contained apartment in a house	12	14
Detached, semi-detached or terraced house	24	39
Other housing arrangements	2	11

Table 3-5. Comparison of the Distribution of Rational
Scale Scores

Scale	Subscale	New York (N=445)		London (N=396)		Kolmogorov Smirnov Test
		Mean	SD	Mean	SD	
Dementia		1.22	2.41	.67	1.59	p < .01
Depression		3.21	3.86	3.17	3.60	NS
Physical illness		5.11	4.59	5.31	3.89	NS
	Arthritis	2.02	1.88	1.98	1.70	NS
	Neurological	.08	.32	.07	.29	NS
	Heart disease	.72	1.13	.87	1.18	NS
	Cancer alert	.24	.61	.36	.63	NS
Perceptual impairment		1.53	2.55	2.19	3.11	p < .01
	Observational items	.22	.52	.24	.51	NS
Immobility		2.68	4.37	2.69	4.14	NS
	Observational items	1.03	1.74	1.17	1.82	NS
Inadequate activities		3.81	2.71	4.58	2.55	p < .01
Current isolation		5.05	2.15	5.19	1.98	NS
Environmental disadvantage		2.61	2.93	2.54	2.15	p < .01
	Observational items	.51	.88	.44	.76	NS
	Crime	.72	1.19	.39	.76	p < .05
Financial disadvantage		.75	1.05	1.04	.47	p < .01

Table 3-6.   Cumulative Frequency Distributions of Rational
              Scale Scores: Dementia

	New York			London		
		Cumulative %'s Progressively				Cumulative %'s Progressively	
Score	N= 445	Higher	Lower	N= 396	Higher	Lower
0	262	58.6	100.0	287	72.5	100.0
1	81	77.2	41.4	53	85.9	27.5
2	34	84.8	22.8	22	91.4	14.1
3	18	88.8	15.2	15	95.2	8.6
4	19	93.1	11.2	7	97.0	4.8
5	5	94.2	6.9	2	97.5	3.0
6	3	94.9	5.8	3	98.2	2.5
7	8	96.6	5.1	0	98.2	1.8
8	3	97.3	3.4	1	98.5	1.8
9	3	98.0	2.7	3	94.2	1.5
10	1	98.2	2.0	2	99.7	.8
11	1	98.4	1.8	1	100.0	.3
12	2	98.9	1.6	0	100.0	0.0
13	3	99.6	1.1	0	100.0	0.0
14	1	99.8	.4	0	100.0	0.0
17	1	100.0	.2	0	100.0	0.0

Table 3-7. Percent Positive Ratings on the Items in
Rational Scale: Dementia

Item Content	Percentage	
	New York (N=445) %	London (N=396) %
* Can't give own name correctly	4	1
Can't repeat rough approximation of interviewer's name	1	1
* Doesn't know age	5	1
Stated age different from that on criterion page	2	1
* Doesn't know year born	10	4
Stated birthday different from that on criterion page	2	1
Uncorrected discrepancy between stated age and birthday	2	1
* Stated birthdate or age obviously wrong	3	1
Doesn't know length of time at present home	5	3
* Doesn't know year moved into home	18	11
Discrepancy between years at address and date moved	3	5

(continues)

Table 3-7. continued

Item Content	Percentage	
	New York (N=445) %	London (N=396) %
*Gives incorrect mailing address	9	3
Doesn't recall name of president/ prime minister	6	9
Doesn't recall name of previous president/prime minister	4	6
States doesn't know day	5	3
Gives wrong day of week or month	3	2
*States doesn't know month	6	1
Gives wrong month	2	1
*States doesn't know year	6	2
Gives wrong year	2	3
*Doesn't recall approximation of interviewer's name	19	6
Perseveration observed - repeats own words	0	0

*The chi square test was used to compare percents with problems in New York City and London by testing for significance at the .05 level. Items with significant differences are indicated with asterisks.

Note: The item frequencies in this and subsequent tables generally indicate the proportion of the population who are deemed to have had the stated problem some time during the past month. The proportions shown in these tables make due allowance for missing data. The exact number of missing responses varies for individual items. The description of each problem is listed in a greatly abbreviated form.

Table 3-8. Cumulative Frequency Distributions of Rational
            Scale Scores: Depression

	New York			London		
		Cumulative %'s Progressively			Cumulative %'s Progressively	
Score	N= 445	Higher	Lower	N= 396	Higher	Lower
0	142	31.8	100.0	102	25.8	100.0
1	68	47.2	68.2	73	44.2	74.2
2	52	58.8	52.8	54	57.8	55.8
3	33	66.2	41.2	31	65.7	42.2
4	25	71.8	33.8	35	74.5	34.3
5	27	78.1	28.2	12	77.5	25.5
6	18	82.1	21.9	25	83.8	22.5
7	14	85.2	17.9	19	88.6	16.2
8	10	87.5	14.8	8	90.7	11.4
9	18	91.5	12.5	7	92.4	9.3
10	10	93.7	8.5	7	94.2	7.6
11	5	94.9	6.3	6	95.7	5.8
12	4	95.7	5.1	8	97.7	4.3
13	7	97.5	4.3	2	98.2	2.3
14	5	98.7	2.5	1	98.5	1.8
15	1	98.9	1.3	2	99.0	1.5
16	3	99.6	1.1	1	99.2	1.0
17	0	99.6	.4	2	99.7	.8
18	2	100.0	.4	0	99.7	.3
19	0	100.0	0.0	1	100.0	.3

Table 3-9. Percent Positive Ratings on the Items in
           Rational Scale: Depression

Item Content	Percentage	
	New York (N=445) %	London (N=396) %
Worries a lot	35	27
Worries about everything	13	18
*Worries bother him	26	15
*Can't stop worrying	17	11
Depressed in last month	28	31
*Has cried	22	13
Has felt like crying	11	13
Depression lasts over few hours	14	16
Time of day depression worst	9	14
Felt life not worth living	11	11
Recently depressed	16	19
Pessimism about future	3	4
Future seems bleak	4	6
Rejected suicide, wished to be dead	8	5
Fleeting suicide thoughts	1	2
Suicide seriously considered	1	0
*Unrealistic self depreciation	1	4
Feels worthless	2	0
Self blame for illness affecting others	1	2
*Self-blame over peccadilloes	3	5

(continues)

Table 3-9. continued

Item Content	Percentage New York (N=445) %	London (N=396) %
*Looks sad, mournful, depressed	16	9
*Sounds gloomy	14	7
Wants to avoid people	4	6
*More irritable lately	6	13
Gets angry with self	9	12
*Awakes early, unable to sleep	11	5
*Difficulty relaxing	12	21
*Restlessness	10	22
*Aches, pains - no physical cause	3	0
Numerous aches and pains - no physical cause	0	0
Preoccupation with somatic complaints	2	1
Says his body is decaying	0	0
*Almost nothing enjoyed	11	6
Subject's judgment of happiness		
Very happy	25	36
Fairly happy	50	50
Not very happy	13	8
Not happy at all	4	2
Long pauses before replying	0	0

*The chi square test was used to compare percents with problems in New York City and London by testing for significance at the .05 level. Items with significant differences are indicated with asterisks.

Table 3-10. Cumulative Frequency Distributions of Rational
            Scale Scores: Total Physical Illness

	New York			London		
		Cumulative %'s Progressively			Cumulative %'s Progressively	
Score	N= 445	Higher	Lower	N= 396	Higher	Lower
0	56	12.5	100.0	36	9.1	100.0
1	54	24.8	87.5	30	16.7	90.9
2	35	32.7	75.2	32	24.7	83.3
3	51	44.1	67.3	51	37.6	75.3
4	45	54.1	55.9	44	48.7	62.4
5	31	61.3	45.9	38	58.3	51.3
6	41	70.5	38.7	31	66.2	41.7
7	28	76.7	29.5	29	73.5	33.8
8	14	79.9	23.3	33	81.8	26.5
9	25	85.7	20.1	23	87.6	18.2
10	9	87.7	14.3	14	91.2	12.4
11	12	90.4	12.3	2	91.7	8.8
12	9	92.4	9.6	3	92.4	8.3
13	11	94.9	7.6	10	94.9	7.6
14	7	96.4	5.1	9	97.2	5.1
15	2	96.9	3.6	4	98.2	2.8
16	3	97.5	3.1	4	99.2	1.8
17	4	98.4	2.5	2	99.7	.8
18	1	98.7	1.6	1	100.0	.3
19	1	98.9	1.3	0	100.0	0.0
21	2	99.3	1.1	0	100.0	0.0
23	1	99.6	.7	0	100.0	0.0
28	1	99.8	.4	0	100.0	0.0
30	1	100.0	.2	0	100.0	0.0

Table 3-11. Percent Positive Ratings on the Items in
             Rational Scale: Total Physical Illness

Item Content	Percentage	
	New York (N=445) %	London (N=396) %
Losing weight due to medical condition	3	4
Difficulty chewing	1	1
Nausea, vomiting	1	3
Wasting despite food intake	1	0
Pain in upper abdomen, related to food intake	18	21
*Above pain persistent over 3 weeks	6	11
Pain in abdomen not easily relieved	5	3
Difficulty swallowing over 3 weeks	2	3
If admits to sleep difficulty-has pain, malaise, itching, breathlessness	9	7
Claims to have blackouts	3	4
Observed impairment of consciousness	0	0
Fainting	4	4
*Fainting without anxiety	15	21
Palpitations on minor exertion	11	11
Prolonged palpitation without exertion	8	7
Palpitations irregular	3	4
If dizzy, fainting, has definite spinning of self	8	7
Faintness preceded by an aura with convulsions, paresis, etc.	0	1
States he has diarrhea	3	2
Pain on bowel movement	1	2
Blood in stool	2	0
Fresh spots of blood	1	2
Blood is black and shiny	1	0
Pain on passing urine	4	3

(continues)

Table 3-11. continued

Item Content	Percentage	
	New York (N=445) %	London (N=396) %
Obstruction to stream	6	5
Often passes a lot of urine	9	9
Often passes a little urine	8	6
Wakes to pass urine	16	18
Recently passed pink urine	1	0
Onset of medical condition coincides with anergia	13	12
Has arthritis	2	1
Has backaches	34	29
Pain, stiffness in joints	37	41
Joint pain in legs	32	34
*Pain in arms or hands	33	26
*Pain in other place	15	8
Migraine	1	1
*Breathlessness	25	32
Breathlessness when lies flat, relieved by pillows	5	8
Chest pain on minor exertion	8	7
Pain relieved by nitroglycerine	6	5
Chest pain on coughing	1	1
Severe unrelieved chest pain	6	4
Pain diagnosed as heart attack	6	3
*Ankle swelling-relieved by elevation	15	21
Steady pressure leaves visible depression on ankles	7	9
*Persistent cough	9	17
Blood in sputum	1	1

(continues)

Table 3-11. continued

Item Content	Percentage New York (N=445) %	London (N=396) %
*Opaque yellow sputum	2	6
Foul-smelling sputum	0	1
Voice recently hoarse	3	4
Persistent chills	2	1
Fever requiring bedrest	1	2
Fever with aftereffects	1	3
Tremor of hands	5	3
States has chronic sore	4	2
Lump in breast	1	1
*Unexplained other lump	2	0
Unexplained bleeding	0	1
Growth requiring operation within last 5 years	6	5
Unsuccessful treatment of malignancy	0	0
Above has effects due to growth	2	1
Has had stroke	6	7
Speaks with slurred speech	1	1
Forgets proper words	0	0
Fracture aftereffects	9	7
Causes some pain	4	5
After effects of an operation	13	11
Observed abnormal movements	1	0
Bent spine	2	1
Twisted limbs	1	1

*The chi square test was used to compare percents with problems in New York City and London by testing for significance at the .05 level. Items with significant differences are indicated with asterisks.

Table 3-12.   Cumulative Frequency Distributions of Rational
              Scale Scores: Total Perceptual Impairment

	New York			London		
		Cumulative %'s			Cumulative %'s	
	N=	Progressively		N=	Progressively	
Score	445	Higher	Lower	396	Higher	Lower
0	264	59.7	100.0	209	52.8	100.0
1	47	70.2	40.3	34	61.4	47.2
2	30	77.0	29.8	25	67.7	38.6
3	30	83.7	23.0	26	74.2	32.3
4	7	85.2	16.3	10	76.8	25.8
5	20	89.7	14.8	21	82.1	23.2
6	12	92.4	10.3	21	87.4	17.9
7	12	95.1	7.6	13	90.7	12.6
8	8	96.9	4.9	14	94.2	9.3
9	7	98.4	3.1	13	97.5	5.8
10	4	99.3	1.6	2	98.0	2.5
11	2	99.8	.7	5	99.2	2.0
12	1	100.0	.2	2	99.7	.8
15	0	100.0	0.0	1	100.0	.3

Table 3-13. Percent Positive Ratings on the Items in
Rational Scale: Total Perceptual Impairment

Item Content	Percentage New York (N=445) %	London (N=396) %
*Difficulty hearing	28	38
*Wears hearing aid at times	4	8
*Observed wearing hearing aid	2	6
*Hearing aid often left off	1	5
*Embarrassed by hearing difficulty	3	10
*Difficulty hearing ordinary conversation	10	18
*Difficulty hearing group conversations	11	22
*Difficulty hearing telephone	4	7
*Difficulty hearing radio	7	14
*Difficulty hearing shopping transactions	2	5
Subject has difficulty hearing interview	14	17
Hears interviewer if shouts	5	3
Trouble seeing	20	17
Can't read regular print	8	8
Can't read telephone directory	11	9
Can't see public signs	4	6
Shopping difficulty due to sight	5	5
Social difficulty due to sight	6	7
Treatment problem due to poor sight	4	4
Trips due to sight	6	5
Doesn't see test items	3	4

*The chi square test was used to compare percents with problems in New York City and London by testing for significance at the .05 level. Items with significant differences are indicated with asterisks.

Table 3-14.   Cumulative Frequency Distributions of Rational
               Scale Scores: Total Immobility

	New York			London		
		Cumulative %'s Progressively			Cumulative %'s Progressively	
Score	N= 445	Higher	Lower	N= 396	Higher	Lower
0	231	51.9	100.0	185	46.7	100.0
1	55	64.2	48.1	50	59.3	53.3
2	20	68.7	35.8	33	67.7	40.7
3	25	74.3	31.3	24	73.7	32.3
4	17	78.1	25.7	18	78.3	26.3
5	15	81.4	21.9	12	81.3	21.7
6	14	84.6	18.6	15	85.1	18.7
7	6	85.9	15.4	9	87.4	14.9
8	9	88.1	14.1	8	89.4	12.6
9	9	90.2	11.9	6	90.9	10.6
10	7	91.7	9.8	9	93.2	9.1
11	6	93.1	8.3	5	94.4	6.8
12	7	94.6	6.9	6	96.0	5.6
13	9	96.6	5.4	5	97.2	4.0
14	2	97.1	3.4	1	97.5	2.8
15	3	97.8	2.9	1	97.7	2.5
16	1	98.0	2.2	2	98.2	2.3
17	3	98.9	2.0	1	98.5	1.8
18	1	99.1	1.1	2	99.0	1.5
19	1	99.3	.9	1	99.2	1.0
20	1	99.6	.7	2	99.7	.8
21	1	99.8	.4	1	100.0	.3
24	1	100.0	.2	0	100.0	0.0

Table 3-15. Percent Positive Ratings on the Items in
Rational Scale: Total Immobility

Item Content	Percentage	
	New York (N=445) %	London (N=396) %
Person not in home prepares meals	4	5
Goes without meals if no prepared	2	0
Difficulty preparing own food	8	7
Dependent on external food service, goes without if can't get there	1	0
Difficulty shopping	17	11
Difficulty ambulating	33	33
Confined to bed during interview	1	0
Confined to wheelchair	0	0
Moves wheelchair without assistance	0	0
*Walks only with assistance	4	1
Walks with walker	2	3
Walks with cane	6	7
Slow getting up to walk	15	17
*Walks slowly, painfully	16	9
Walks bent	7	10
*Uses wheelchair outdoors	1	3
Needs assistance outdoors	8	6
Can't manage one flight of stairs	8	7
Can't manage trains, buses	13	15

(continues)

Table 3-15. continued

Item Content	Percentage New York (N=445) %	London (N=396) %
Can't manage heavy doors	9	12
Occasionally trips	8	9
Can't cross roads	9	8
Can't manage one level block	6	5
Can't manage 1-2 blocks	14	11
*Difficulty reaching for toes	9	17
Can't reach toes at all	5	8
Difficulty lifting arms overhead	5	6
Can't reach dominant hand in back	3	3
Can't rotate dominant arm	2	1
Limited movement of arm	1	1
Limited movement of leg	2	2
Problem using toilet alone	1	1
Problem using shower	13	15
Difficulty doing chores	24	21
*Subject looks frail	8	11
Subject looks emaciated	1	1
Subject looks physically ill	5	5
Subject looks seriously ill	1	1

*The chi square test was used to compare percents with problems in New York City and London by testing for significance at the .05 level. Items with significant differences are indicated with asterisks.

Table 3-16.   Cumulative Frequency Distributions of Rational
              Scale Scores: Inadequate Activities

	New York			London		
		Cumulative %'s Progressively			Cumulative %'s Progressively	
Score	N= 445	Higher	Lower	N= 396	Higher	Lower
0	35	7.8	100.0	12	3.0	100.0
1	48	18.8	92.2	31	10.9	97.0
2	67	33.8	81.2	44	22.0	89.1
3	93	54.6	66.2	57	36.4	78.0
4	65	69.1	45.4	59	51.3	63.6
5	43	79.0	30.9	62	66.9	48.7
6	22	83.9	21.0	48	79.0	33.1
7	19	88.1	16.1	31	86.9	21.0
8	17	91.9	11.9	22	92.4	13.1
9	11	94.6	8.1	16	96.5	7.6
10	14	97.8	5.4	7	98.2	3.5
11	8	99.6	2.2	3	99.0	1.8
12	0	99.6	.4	1	99.2	1.0
13	2	100.0	.4	3	100.0	.8

Table 3-17.   Percent Positive Ratings on the Items in
              Rational Scale: Inadequate Activities

Item Content	Percentage	
	New York (N=445) %	London (N=396) %
Not going out more a problem	9	8
Not out as often as needs	12	8
Not out as often as wants to	22	19
No letters received	36	35
Has had no visitors	16	12
*Had less than 3 personal telephone chats	20	37
Does almost no shopping	43	47
Sits around due to lack of energy	15	19
Spends little time at recreation	10	7
*Club member	46	39
*Is a club member and has attended meeting in past month	21	26
*Is a member of religious congregation	53	39
*Is a member but does not attend religious services regularly	65	87
Does no household chores alone	47	43

*The chi square test was used to compare percents with problems in New York City and London by testing for significance at the .05 level. Items with significant differences are indicated with asterisks.

Table 3-18. Cumulative Frequency Distributions of Rational
Scale Scores: Current Isolation

	New York			London		
		Cumulative %'s			Cumulative %'s	
	N=	Progressively		N=	Progressively	
Score	445	Higher	Lower	396	Higher	Lower
0	8	1.8	100.0	3	.8	100.0
1	14	4.9	98.2	16	4.8	99.2
2	44	15.0	95.1	40	14.9	95.2
3	44	24.8	85.0	40	25.0	85.1
4	80	43.0	75.2	70	42.7	75.0
5	66	57.7	57.0	70	60.4	57.3
6	85	76.7	42.3	86	82.1	39.6
7	43	86.6	33.3	35	90.9	17.9
8	39	95.3	13.4	26	97.5	9.1
9	18	99.3	4.7	8	99.5	2.5
10	3	100.0	.7	2	100.0	.5

The scale scores in this table are inverted (by scoring 2+
as 0, 1 as 1, and 0 as 2) so that higher scores refer to
fewer contacts or more isolation.

Table 3-19.   Mean Score on the Items in Rational Scale[a]
              of Current Isolation

| | Mean Score | |
Item Content	New York (N=445)	London (N=396)
Number of children seen this month	1.33	1.32
*Number of siblings seen this month	.53	.67
*Number of relatives seen this month	1.49	1.07
*Number of friends seen this month	1.74	1.42
*Number of clubs respondent belongs to	.64	.49

[a]Items in this Table are described as number of social
contacts. The item data are given as mean scores of social
contacts. Higher numbers mean more contacts. However, the
scale scores shown in Table 3-18 are inverted (by scoring 2 +
as 0, 1 as 1, and 0 as 2) so that higher scale scores refer to
fewer contacts or more isolation.

*The t-test was used to compare means on the items between the
two cities. Significant differences at the .05 level or
higher are indicated with asterisks.

Table 3-20.   Cumulative Frequency Distributions of Rational
              Scale Scores: Total Environmental Disadvantage

	New York			London		
		Cumulative %'s			Cumulative %'s	
	N=	Progressively		N=	Progressively	
Score	445	Higher	Lower	396	Higher	Lower
0	133	30.0	100.0	60	15.2	100.0
1	70	45.9	70.0	86	36.9	84.8
2	61	59.7	54.1	94	60.6	63.1
3	47	70.2	40.3	52	73.7	39.4
4	40	79.2	29.8	36	82.8	26.3
5	25	84.8	20.8	26	89.4	17.2
6	25	90.4	15.2	17	93.7	10.6
7	19	94.6	9.6	10	96.2	6.3
8	6	96.0	5.4	11	99.0	3.8
9	2	96.4	4.0	1	99.2	1.0
10	5	97.5	3.6	2	99.7	.8
11	3	98.2	2.5	1	100.0	.3
12	2	98.7	1.8	0	100.0	0.0
13	3	99.3	1.3	0	100.0	0.0
14	1	99.6	.7	0	100.0	0.0
16	1	99.8	.4	0	100.0	0.0
19	1	100.0	.2	0	100.0	0.0

Table 3-21.   Percent Positive Ratings on the Items in Rational
               Scale: Total Environmental Disadvantage

Item Content*	Percentage	
	New York (N=445) %	London (N=396) %
*No telephone	7	41
*Telephone access difficult	3	16
Noise a problem for sleeping	3	3
No bedroom a problem	1	0
High noise level a problem	9	9
Inadequate lighting	1	1
*Not enough heat	13	4
*Inadequate heat creates problems	11	2
*Access to home difficult - no elevator	12	4
Access difficulty - elevator broken	2	2
Access difficulty a problem	6	4
*No refrigerator	1	10
*No refrigerator a problem	0	4
Has refrigerator - causes problems	2	2
No stove	0	1
No stove a problem	0	0
Problem related to stove	4	0
*No toilet in apartment	0	8
Toilet often not working	1	0
Problem getting to toilet - unsafe	0	0
*No bathing facilities in apartment	0	10

(continues)

Table 3-21. continued

Item Content*	Percentage	
	New York (N=445) %	London (N=396) %
Bathing facilities not often working	2	2
High crime rate in area	26	24
House broken into in last year	4	3
House broken into since age 65	9	6
*Crime involving self	4	1
*Crime involving self since age 65	10	2
Crime involving personal injury	2	1
*Crime involving personal injury since age 65	4	1
*Feels apartment unsafe	13	3
Rats and mice in dwelling	6	5
Rats a problem	3	1
Deterioration of area	38	34
*Problem with landlord	14	8
Condition of living unit: poor	7	3
Condition of building: poor	13	8
Condition of area: poor	23	19
Type of housing on block: multiple occupancy	9	12
Type of neighborhood: less than half residential	7	3

*The chi square test was used to compare percents with problems in New York City and London by testing for significance at the .05 level. Items with significant differences are indicated with asterisks.

Table 3-22.   Cumulative Frequency Distributions of Rational
              Scale Scores: Financial Disadvantage

	New York			London		
Score	N= 445	Cumulative %'s Progressively Higher	Lower	N= 396	Cumulative %'s Progressively Higher	Lower
0	252	56.6	100.0	25	6.3	100.0
1	109	81.2	43.4	343	92.9	93.7
2	31	88.4	12.8	16	97.0	7.1
3	47	98.9	11.6	12	100.0	3.0
4	5	100.0	1.1	0	100.0	0.0

Table 3-23.   Percent Positive Ratings on the Items in
              Rational Scale: Financial Disadvantage

Item Content	Percentage	
	New York (N=445) %	London (N=396) %
*Can't afford food	2	0
Can't afford transport to doctor	1	1
Income below median in each city	Not relevant for cross-national comparison	
*Subject describes financial problem	19	7
*Examiner has determined existence of financial problem	19	5

*The chi square test was used to compare percents with
problems in New York City and London by testing for significance
at the .05 level.   Items with significant differences are
indicated with asterisks.

Table 3-24. Mean Rational Score of Dementia by Subsample

| | New York | | London | |
Subsample	Mean Score	N	Mean Score	N
1	1.7	88	.7	88
2	1.1	95	.5	74
3	1.3	105	.4	74
4	1.1	81	.7	66
5	.9	76	.9	94
Total	1.2	445	.7	396

Table 3-25. Overlap of Dementia Mean Rational Scores by
Subsample

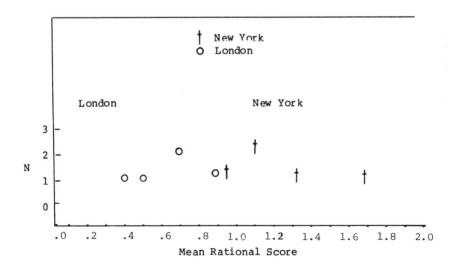

Table 3-26. Mean Rational Score of Depression by Subsample

Subsample	New York Mean Score	N	London Mean Score	N
1	3.5	88	3.0	88
2	3.7	95	3.2	74
3	2.6	105	3.0	74
4	2.8	81	3.2	66
5	3.5	76	3.3	94
Total	3.2	445	3.2	396

Table 3-27 appears on pages 96–97.

Table 3-28. Summary of Intercorrelations Among Rational Scales in New York (N=445) and London (N=396)

Pearson Product Moment Correlations

		Depression	Physical illness	Perceptual impairment	Immobility	Inadequate activities	Current isolation	Environmental disadvantage	Financial disadvantage
Dementia	New York	.14	.14	.14	.33	.28	.13	.09	.18
	London	-.01	-.05	-.01	.30	.25	.09	.01	.03
Depression	New York		.47	.17	.42	.40	.04	.18	.26
	London		.37	.13	.15	.21	.01	.21	.05
Physical illness	New York			.15	.52	.39	.08	.28	.34
	London			.22	.33	.24	.02	.20	.01
Perceptual impairment	New York				.29	.28	.01	.01	.08
	London				.13	.10	-.01	.00	-.07
Immobility	New York					.65	-.15	.09	.27
	London					.56	-.13	.14	-.03
Inadequate activities	New York						.34	.14	.20
	London						.14	.08	.03
Current isolation	New York							.16	.12
	London							.04	.10
Environmental disadvantage	New York								.38
	London								.14

Note: For n's of 396 and over, in this and subsequent tables, all correlations greater than .08 are significant at the .05 level.

Table 3-27. Comparison of the Means and Standard Deviations
of Homogeneous Scales of Health and Social Problems

	New York (N=445) Mean	SD*	London (N=396) Mean	SD*	Kolmogorov Smirnov Test
Health Problems					
Organic Brain Syndrome	1.44	1.98	.86	1.48	p < .01
Depression	4.30	4.66	4.38	4.47	p < .05
Suspiciousness	.10	.43	.21	.63	ns
Subjective Memory	1.27	1.87	1.20	1.77	ns
Retirement Dissatisfaction	.87	1.55	.50	1.18	ns
Sleep Disorder	1.48	1.72	1.21	1.66	p < .05
Somatic Symptoms	3.06	3.61	3.23	3.26	p < .05
Heart Disorder	1.36	2.19	1.13	2.11	ns
Stroke Effects	.26	1.13	.27	1.11	ns
Cancer	.45	1.04	.30	.93	ns
Respiratory Symptoms	.80	1.16	1.28	1.38	p < .01
Arthritis	2.69	2.64	2.43	2.13	ns
Leg Swelling	.88	1.59	1.22	1.66	p < .01
Malnutrition	.67	1.48	.86	1.77	ns
Hearing Disorder	1.05	2.07	1.79	2.76	p < .01
Vision Disorder	.67	1.93	.69	1.97	ns
Hypertension	.68	1.21	.52	1.12	ns
Ambulation Problems	3.18	5.16	3.27	4.65	ns
Activity Limitation	4.47	7.08	4.81	6.28	ns
Dependency	3.57	4.66	4.02	4.36	ns
Health Limitations	1.79	2.90	1.91	3.06	ns

(continues)

Table 3-27. continued

	New York (N=445)		London (N=396)		Kolmogorov Smirnov Test
	Mean	SD*	Mean	SD*	
Social Problems					
Financial Hardship	.76	1.49	.33	.86	p < .01
Disatisfaction with Neighborhood	1.05	1.35	.97	1.24	ns
Fear of Crime	1.90	2.70	1.06	1.94	p < .01
Housing Problem	1.04	1.79	.64	1.23	p < .05
Isolation from Family	4.62	3.37	4.75	3.30	ns
Social Isolation Problems	8.06	3.90	10.82	3.87	p < .01
Subjective Isolation Problems	1.79	1.98	1.96	1.98	ns
Family Contact Problems	1.06	1.94	1.42	2.08	p < .01
Response Styles					
General Complaining	6.07	5.20	6.15	4.70	ns
Denial	.31	.91	.15	.72	ns

*Standard deviation for the scale.

Table 3-29.   Intercorrelations between Rational Scales and
              Age, Sex, Monthly Income

| | Pearson Product Moment Correlations | | | | | |
| | New York (N=445) | | | London (N=396) | | |
Scale	Age	Sex[1]	Monthly Income	Age	Sex[1]	Monthly Income
Dementia	.25	.11	.10	.29	.14	-.09
Depression	.02	.12	-.05	-.09	.12	-.03
Physical illness	-.01	.10	.01	.09	.04	-.00
Perceptual impairment	.22	-.10	.01	.28	.02	.02
Immobility	.31	.10	.07	.37	.09	-.07
Inadequate activities	.23	-.02	-.08	.19	-.11	-.02
Current isolation	.04	-.02	-.08	.18	-.08	-.00
Environmental disadvantage	-.07	.09	-.13	.04	.02	-.08
Financial disadvantage	.04	.17	-.26[2]	.06	.01	-.17[2]

[1]Positive correlations indicate that females score higher
on the scale, negative correlations indicate that males
score higher.

[2]Monthly income below median is an item on the Financial
Disadvantage scale, see Table 3-23.

Table 3-30. Intercorrelations between Rational Scales and
            Education and Occupation

Scale	New York (N=445) Education	Occupation	London (N=396) Education	Occupation
Dementia	-.19	-.19	-.14	-.12
Depression	-.07	.02	-.03	.01
Physical illness	-.07	-.02	-.10	-.05
Perceptual impairment	-.03	.06	-.03	.01
Immobility	-.05	.00	-.09	-.05
Inadequate activities	-.10	-.01	-.16	-.14
Current Isolation	.06	-.03	.13	.10
Environmental disadvantage	-.09	-.14	-.04	-.12
Financial disadvantage	-.17	-.14	-.04	-.01

For this table both education and occupation were collapsed as
shown below.

education scored   0 = < 8th grade   1 = 8th grade +

occupation scored 0 = blue collar   1 = white collar,
                     or service   professional

Table 3-31 appears on pages 102-103.

Table 3-32. Table of Overlap between Screening Criteria for Depression and Dementia

NEW YORK

| | Unique to this criterion | Overlap with | | | Total |
		Rational scale 6+	Latent class	Global Impairment	
(a) rational scale 6+ on depression or dementia	15	X	66	86	115
(b) latent class probability $\geq$ .90 for depression or dementia	10	66	X	55	83
(c) global psychiatric impairment $\geq$ 4	38	86	55	X	124

Unduplicated total = 172

LONDON

| | Unique to this criterion | Overlap with | | | Total |
		Rational scale 6+	Latent class	Global Impairment	
(a) rational scale 6+ on depression or dementia	18	X	66	40	87
(b) latent class probability $\geq$ .90 for depression or dementia	17	66	X	40	86
(c) global psychiatric impairment $\geq$ 4	10	40	40	X	53

Unduplicated total = 142

Table 3-33. Reliability of Pervasive Dementia Diagnosis

| | | Rater A | | |
		Not Pervasive Dementia	Pervasive Dementia	Total
Rater B	Not Pervasive Dementia	100	3	103
	Pervasive Dementia	6	15	21
	Total:	106	18	N=124

Po = .93
Pc = .73
*Kappa = .73

*Kappa is a statistic which measures the extent of agreement between raters, corrected for the amount of agreement which might be expected by chance alone. It varies from 0 (no more agreement than would be expected by chance) to 1 (complete agreement).

Table 3-34. Reliability of Pervasive Depression Diagnosis

| | | Rater A | | |
		Not Pervasive Depression	Pervasive Depression	Total
Rater B	Not Pervasive Depression	86	5	91
	Pervasive Depression	7	26	33
	Total:	93	31	N=124

Po = .90
Pc = .62
*Kappa = .75

*Kappa is a statistic which measures the extent of agreement between raters, corrected for the amount of agreement which might be expected by chance alone. It varies from 0 (no more agreement than would be expected by chance) to 1 (complete agreement).

Table 3-31. Mean Scores on Selected Rational Scales by Race, Marital Status, and Living Arrangements

New York

Scale	Race White (N=378)	Race Non White* (N=67)	Marital Status Married (N=206)	Marital Status Unmarried (N=233)	Living Arrangement Not Alone (N=289)	Living Arrangement Alone (N=134)
Dementia	1.04	2.28***	1.00	1.41[1]	1.24	1.19
Depression	3.24	3.06	2.93	3.48	3.16	3.31
Physical illness	5.01	5.72	4.96	5.32	4.95	5.44
Perceptual impairment	1.62	1.06[1]	1.44	1.64	1.49	1.61
Immobility	2.67	2.67	2.09	3.12*	2.55	2.90
Inadequate activities	3.81	3.87	3.88	3.76	4.00	3.47*
Current isolation	4.93	5.71**	5.29	4.84*	5.10	5.00

London

Scale	Race White (N=391)	Race Non White (N=3)	Marital Status Married (N=185)	Marital Status Unmarried (N=208)	Living Arrangement Not Alone (N=258)	Living Arrangement Alone (N=138)
Dementia	.67	.57	.44	.88**	.71	.58
Depression	3.16	4.14	3.12	3.22	2.91	3.65[1]
Physical illness	5.35	3.57	5.21	5.44	5.00	5.88*
Perceptual impairment	2.20	2.29	1.78	2.55*	1.91	2.71*
Immobility	2.75	.86[2]	1.94	3.43***	2.36	3.36*
Inadequate activities	4.60	4.43	4.66	4.54	4.83	4.14*
Current isolation	5.18	6.20	5.01	5.33	5.09	5.31

Table 3-31.

New York

Scale	Race		Marital Status		Living Arrangement	
	White (N=378)	Non White* (N=67)	Married (N=206)	Unmarried (N=233)	Not Alone (N=289)	Alone (N=134)
Environmental disadvantage	2.10	5.52***	2.35	2.89[1]	2.38	3.06*
Financial disadvantage	.63	1.42***	.48	.99***	.68	.88[1]

London

Scale	Race		Marital Status		Living Arrangement	
	White (N=391)	Non White (N=3)	Married (N=185)	Unmarried (N=208)	Not Alone (N=258)	Alone (N=138)
Environmental disadvantage	2.53	3.71	2.25	2.83**	2.18	3.22***
Financial disadvantage	1.03	1.29	1.02	1.05	1.02	1.06

* Non-white includes blacks, Hispanic and other.

F test was computed comparing mean scores for the two categories of race, marital status, living arrangement.

   * F ratio significant, p < .05
  ** F ratio significant, p < .01
 *** F ratio significant, p < .001

The degrees of freedom is always $N_1 + N_2 - 2$

[1] F ratio just misses significance, p < .10

[2] Despite large difference in means, this difference is not significant due to small sample size of nonwhite group.

NOTE: Number of subjects in subcategories do not always add up to the total samples because of missing data. Marital status was unknown in six subjects in New York and three in London. Race was uncoded for two subjects in London, and living arrangement was uncoded for 22 subjects in New York.

Table 3-35.   Point (Past Month) Prevalence Rates of Pervasive
              Depression and Dementia in New York and London

| | Point Prevalence Rates | | | |
| | New York | | London | |
	N	%	N	%
Pervasive depression	58	13.0	49	12.4
Pervasive dementia	22	4.9	9	2.3
Neither	365	82.0	338	85.3
Total	445	99.9	396	100.0

Table 3-37.   Correlations of Demographic Variables with the
              Rational Scale of Dementia

| | Pearson Product Moment Correlations | |
Demographic variable*	New York	London
Age	.25	.29
Race	-.17	.02
Sex	.11	.14
Education	-.19	-.14
Occupation	-.19	-.12
Marital Status	-.09	-.13

*All demographic variables except age are dichotomized, with
white, female, > 8 years education, white collar, professional
occupation, and married scoring 1; and non-white, male, $\leq$ 8
years education, blue collar and unskilled workers, and
unmarried scoring 0.

Table 3-36. Point (Past Month) Prevalence Rates of Depression and Dementia by Various Indicators

Criteria	Prevalence Rates		Ratio of
	New York	London	New York to London
Depression			
Pervasive depression	13.0%	12.4%	1.04
6 or more on rational scale of depression	22.0%	22.5%	.97
Latent class probability over .90	22.0%	17.9%	1.22
Manic-depressive-depressive disorder*	2.5%	1.3%	1.9
Dementia			
Pervasive Dementia	4.9%	2.3%	2.13
6 or more on rational scale of dementia	5.8%	2.5%	2.32
Latent class probability over .90	10.6%	4.3%	2.46
Alzheimer's (senile) dementia*	3.9%	2.0%	1.95

*See Appendices I and II for definition of these disorders in terms of study criteria.

Table 3-38. A Comparison of Rational Scale Scores of
Dementia in London and New York Controlling
for Age and Sex

Females
only: Numbers of persons with scores of 6 or more on
the rational scale of dementia

| | New York | | London | | | |
| | | | Unadjusted | | Adjusted to equal New York age distribution | |
Age Groups	N	Score 6+	N	Score 6+	N	Score 6+
65-69	81	2	76	0	81	0
70-74	75	3	78	0	75	0
75-79	60	5	46	2	60	3
80+	50	10	48	8	50	8
Total	266	20	248	10	266	11

Males
only: Numbers of persons with scores of 6 or more on
the rational scale of dementia

| | New York | | London | | | |
| | | | Unadjusted | | Adjusted to equal New York age distribution | |
Age Groups	N	Score 6+	N	Score 6+	N	Score 6+
65-69	61	0	49	0	61	0
70-74	48	1	41	0	48	0
75-79	35	2	34	0	35	0
80+	33	3	14	0	33	0
Total	177	6	138	0	177	0

_____ Figures in framed boxes allow age and sex controlled
_____ cross-national comparison of rates of dementia

Table 3-39. Cumulative Rational Scores of Dementia in New
York and and London, Adjusted to Allow for Assumed
Differences in Education

Cumulative error score on rational scale of dementia	New York			London
	Unadjusted	Discounting one error	Discounting two errors	
0	100.0	100.0	100.0	100.0
1	41.4	22.8	15.2	27.5
2	22.8	15.2	11.2	14.1
3	15.2	11.2	6.9	8.6
4	11.2	6.9	5.8	4.8
5	6.9	5.8	5.1	3.0
6	5.8	5.1	3.4	2.5
7	5.1	3.4	2.7	1.8
8	3.4	2.7	2.0	1.0
9	2.7	2.0	1.8	1.5
10	2.0	1.8	1.6	.8
11	1.8	1.6	1.1	.3
12	1.6	1.1	.4	.0
13	1.1	.4	.2	
14	.4	.2	.2	
15	.2	.2	.2	
16	.2	.2		
17	.2			

108

Table 3-40. Age and Sex Differences for Selected Rational Scales for New York and London Samples

Mean Rational Scale Scores

New York

Scale	Males				Females			
	65-69 yr (N=61)	70-74 (N=48)	75-79 yr (N=35)	80+ yr (N=33)	65-69 yr (N=81)	70-74 yr (N=75)	75-79 yr (N=60)	80+ yr (N=50)
Dementia	.31	.50	1.20	1.94***	1.07	.76	1.70	2.98***
Depression	2.62	1.60	2.26	5.06***	3.63	3.80	3.27	3.44
Physical illness	4.74	3.27	4.86	5.78	5.38	5.16	5.72	5.98
Perceptual impairment	.87	1.58	1.74	3.91***	.60	1.57	1.65	1.94**
Immobility	1.33	.98	2.51	5.12***	1.69	2.29	3.17	6.08***
Inadequate activities	3.61	3.60	4.29	4.91*	3.31	3.01	4.00	5.14***

London

Scale	Males				Females			
	65-69 yr (N=49)	70-74 yr (N=41)	75-79 yr (N=34)	80+ yr (N=14)	65-69 yr (N=76)	70-74 yr (N=78)	75-79 yr (N=48)	80+ yr (N=56)
Dementia	.55	.24	.24	.36	.38	.47	.92	1.86***
Depression	2.73	2.07	2.94	2.50	3.64	4.24	3.15	2.54
Physical illness	4.63	4.17	5.71	7.79*	5.21	5.27	5.90	5.54
Perceptual impairment	1.16	1.78	2.79	4.93***	1.79	1.37	2.56	3.71***
Immobility	1.57	1.98	2.88	3.79	1.00	2.06	4.46	5.59***
Inadequate activities	5.20	4.83	4.82	4.86	3.45	4.08	5.00	5.55***

(continues)

Table 3-40. continued

Mean Rational Scale Scores

| | New York | | | | | | | | London | | | | | | | |
| | Males | | | | Females | | | | Males | | | | Females | | | |
Scale	65-69 yr (N=61)	70-74 yr (N=48)	75-79 yr (N=35)	80+ yr (N=33)	65-69 yr (N=81)	70-74 yr (N=75)	75-79 yr (N=60)	80+ yr (N=50)	65-69 yr (N=49)	70-74 yr (N=41)	75-79 yr (N=34)	80+ yr (N=14)	65-69 yr (N=76)	70-74 yr (N=78)	75-79 yr (N=48)	80+ yr (N=56)
Current isolation	4.77	4.96	6.03	4.94	5.16	4.93	4.63	5.40	5.14	5.29	6.00	5.29	4.54	4.69	6.15	5.41
Environmental disadvantage	2.33	2.27	3.09	1.48	3.42	2.23	3.03	2.54	2.80	2.34	2.12	2.79	2.20	2.71	2.52	2.91
Financial disadvantage	.54	.25	.66	.82*	.79	.95	.83	1.04	.98	1.05	1.03	1.07	1.05	.95	1.15	1.07

F test was computed comparing mean scores for each age category

*F ratio significant, p < .05
**F ratio significant, p < .01
***F ratio significant, p < .001

df_1 = number of categories - 1 $df_2 = N_1 + N_2 + \ldots N_9 - 1$

Table 3-41. Information Required for Judging Personal Time
Dependency

Provider Services	Disabilities
Medical or nursing consultation. Treatment or prevention of pressure sores. Nursing of wounds. Tube or intravenous feeding. Cleaning of incontinence. Toilet training. Care of catheter, diaper nursing.	Physiological disability: Disturbance of automatic movements such as swallowing, protective reflexes, shifting movements, control of bladder and bowel, healing processes, etc.
Assistance or supervision in bathing, grooming, walking, transferring, feeding, routine care of feet or fingernails.	Disability in activities of daily living: Disturbance of coordinated movements such as feeding, standing, moving inside residence, managing stairs, moving about outside residence, bathing, dressing, grooming, effort intolerance, etc.
Reminders and supervision to avoid dangers or find way around. Advice on business, finances, accounting, budgeting. Alerting and warnings of impending or actual illness, fainting or falling.	Faulty or inconsistent awareness: Disturbance of awareness, anticipation, or orientation with an inability to avoid simple dangers, remain aware of basic needs, find way around, be alert to or remember episodes of falling or illness, maintain consciousness, make plans for the future, etc.
Shopping, planning meals, following diet plan, preparing food, cooking. Housekeeping tasks, laundry. Errands, correspondence, reading. Escort for outside excursions. Managing cash (not budget). Supervising medications or nursing instructions.	Disability in instrumental activities of daily living: Disturbance of complex tasks such as household cleaning chores, shopping, cooking and preparing meals, managing cash, writing and reading, following medication or nursing regimen, using public transport, etc.

(continues)

Table 3-41. continued

Provider Services	Disabilities
Encouragement or persuasion to take exercise, carry out tasks and engage in activities. Companionship, sitting services.	Inadequate emotional autonomy: Disturbance of self-regulation and self-sufficiency with an inability to tolerate being alone, maintain motivation, take needed exercise, maintain interests and activities, etc.
Advocacy and intermediation for subject as an individual. Summoning medical or social help as needed. Sheltering from public contact. Protecting from repercussions of social behavior, governing social relations.	Inadequate social initiative: Inability to take required or desired social action such as communicating, or obtaining medical help when needed, obtaining physical assistance when needed (e.g., chairs, walkers, rails), tolerating contact with the public, maintaining minimal decorum and manners; making, breaking and maintaining interpersonal relationships.

Table 3-42. Level of Agreement in Diagnosing Personal Time Dependency

			Rater B		
			Not PTD	PTD	Total
	Not PTD		59	6	65
Rater A					
	PTD		5	34	39
			—	—	—
		Total:	64	40	N=104

$$P_o = .89$$
$$P_c = .53$$
$$*Kappa = .78$$

*Kappa is a statistic which measures the extent of agreement between raters, corrected for the amount of agreement which might be expected by chance alone. It varies from 0 (no more agreement than would be expected by chance) to 1 (complete agreement).

Table 3-43. An Indicator Scale of Personal Time Dependency

Indicator	Corrected Item-Whole Correlation Coefficient**	
	New York	London
Unable to perform essential tasks	.56	.38
Depends on others for excursions	.72	.65
Physical difficulty getting to doctor	.44	.57
Can't care for essential needs	.49	.50
Can't ambulate without assistance	.60	.46
Can't manage essential task because of ambulation	.64	.55
Health limits mobility	.68	.56
Health limits carrying packages	.72	.57
Poor vision impedes tasks	.36	.19
Doesn't know phone number	.42	.19
Problems handling business by self	.57	.28
Problems dressing by self	.62	.43
Problems grooming self	.58	.34
Problems grooming due to physical disabilities	.62	.44
Does almost no chores by self	.49	.55
Difficulty doing housework by self	.64	.63
Problems doing the laundry	.46	.37
Couldn't survive without help	.70	.71
Hasn't been out in past week	.46	.52
Can't prepare own meals	.59	.48
Has help with shopping	.51	.57
Because of difficulty spouse does shopping	.42	.55
Can't do shopping	.78	.74
Can't cross streets	.67	.48
Difficulty cutting toenails	.56	.34
Health limits light chores	.66	.54
Problems using bath by self	.68	.45
Could not manage chores without help	.74	.76
Because of difficulty spouse does chores	.64	.60

Scale Statistics

Cronbach's alpha, a measure of internal consistency	.94	.92
Mean	5.24	5.26
Standard Deviation	6.53	5.73

**The item-whole correlations have been adjusted to eliminate the spurious association caused by the fact that the item is also part of the scale.

Table 3-44. Demographic Characteristics of Personal
Time Dependents

	Percent Dependent		Total N's	
Characteristics	New York 30%	London 31%	New York (N=445)	London (N=396)
Marital Status				
Never married	13	23	(31)	(43)
Divorced/Separated	18	50	(22)	(10)
Widowed	36	41	(181)	(155)
Married	26	24	(206)	(185)
Missing data			(5)	(3)
Living Arrangements				
Lives alone	25	33	(134)	(138)
Lives with others	31	30	(291)	(258)
Missing data			(20)	(0)
Sex				
Male	24	27	(177)	(138)
Female	33	34	(268)	(258)
Religion				
Protestant	34	30	(92)	(301)
Jewish	30	31	(146)	(13)
Catholic	27	38	(166)	(40)
Other	30	32	(20)	(37)
Missing data			(21)	(5)

(continues)

Table 3-44. continued

Characteristics	Percent Dependent		Total N's	
	New York 30%	London 31%	New York (N=445)	London (N=396)
Race				
White	29	31	(378)	(391)
Black	37	33	(44)	(3)
Hispanic	50	–	(18)	
Other	25	–	(4)	
Missing data			(1)	(2)
Nativity				
Immigrant	31	32	(265)	(40)
Native Born	29	31	(173)	(355)
Missing data			(7)	(1)
Neighborhood Condition				
Poor	37	27	(89)	(75)
Average	28	30	(233)	(230)
*Good	22	42	(88)	(79)
Missing data			(35)	(12)

*The chi square test was used to compare percents dependent in New York City and London by testing for significance at the .05 level. Items with significant differences are indicated with asterisks.

Table 3-45. Relationship between Age and Personal Time Depende
New York and London (in percents)

Age	Percent Dependent			
	New York 30%	N 132	London 31%	N 124
65-69	17	24	18	23
70-74	24	29	19	24
75-79	34	32	28	35
80+	53	46	34	42
Unknown	--	1	--	--

Table 3-46. The Relationship Between Personal Time Dependency
and Indices of Psychiatric, Medical and Social
Conditions (Mean Scores on Rational Scales)

	Inde-pendent	Levels of Dependence Limited Home Care	Adult Home	Nursing Home	All Dependents
Possible Causes					
Dementia					
New York	.65	1.40	2.02	4.35	2.57**
London	.32	.83	1.10	3.11	1.44**
Arthritis					
New York	1.88	2.11	2.64	2.28	2.35**
London	1.86	2.57	2.14	1.85	2.24**
Heart					
New York	.59	.79	1.22	1.07	1.03**
London	.13	.98	1.16	1.44	1.15**
Neurological					
New York	.01	.14	.18	.37	.23**
London	.04	.06	.16	.30	.15**
Physical					
New York	4.23	5.52	7.35	8.72	7.18**
London	4.65	6.66	6.70	7.00	6.75**
Immobility					
New York	.81	3.86	7.35	10.20	7.12**
London	.88	3.95	7.32	10.22	6.68**
Perceptual					
New York	1.05	2.52	2.66	2.79	2.66**
London	1.69	3.21	3.86	2.37	3.29**
Possible Effects					
Depression					
New York	2.58	4.11	4.31	5.72	4.70**
London	2.73	4.48	3.64	4.44	4.14**
Inadequate Activities					
New York	2.80	4.68	6.44	7.58	6.23**
London	3.67	5.08	7.04	8.33	6.58**
Current Isolation					
New York	5.13	4.56	5.04	3.90	4.51**
London	4.99	4.26	4.78	4.07	4.43**

(continues)

Table 3-46. continued

	Inde- pendent	Levels of Dependence			All Dependents
		Limited Home Care	Adult Home	Nursing Home	
Possible Disadvantages					
Financial					
New York	.62	.75	1.28	1.12	1.05**
London	1.03	1.00	1.06	1.15	1.06
Crime					
New York	.74	.93	.62	.40	.65
London	.40	.47	.32	.33	.38
Environment					
New York	2.46	2.93	3.20	2.70	2.95
London	.46	.26	.38	.74	.41
Total N's					
New York	(313)	(44)	(45)	(43)	(132)
London	(272)	(47)	(50)	(27)	(124)

F ratio for one-way analysis of variance showed significant differences in mean scores for dependent versus independent sample.

  *F ratio significant, p $\leq$ .05
 **F ratio significant, p $\leq$ .01

Table 3-47.   The Frequency of Pervasive Depression in Association with Personal Time Dependency*

Pervasive Depression	Independent				Personal Time Dependent			
	New York		London		New York		London	
	100%	(313)	100%	(273)	100%	(132)	100%	(124)
Absent	89%	(275)	90%	(247)	84%	(111)	81%	(101)
Present	12%	(38)	10%	(26)	16%	(21)	19%	(23)

*The association between depression and PTD is examined in Table 3-47 and Figure 3-5. In the former, diagnosis is used as the indicator of depression, in the latter, all types and levels of depression are taken into account including demoralization. Thus the two tables are not comparable.

Section IV
Service Utilization

This section compares the use of health and social services by the elderly in New York and London; and also presents some data on self-help practices of these populations. It should be kept in mind that these data were reported by the subjects or close informants and were not verified from other sources; an exception being the use of medications.

In this section we discuss services used by:

(1) a cross-section of the elderly,

(2) the elderly with dementia or depression, and

(3) the dependent elderly.

In 1, for the sake of brevity, we restrict the data largely to those showing significant cross-national differences. The chi squares were computed with 1 degree of freedom; differences were significant at the $p < .05$ level. In 2 and 3 the data show both differences and similarities.

1. COMPARISON OF SERVICES USED BY A CROSS-SECTION OF THE ELDERLY

A. Medical and Non-medical Health Services

The vast majority of the elderly in London are beneficiaries of the National Health Service, while in New York, Medicare is the most commonly reported third party source of payment for health services. The National Health Services is an organization of services as well as a method of financing; in this sense, the Health Insurance Plan (HIP) program, a prepaid health maintenance organization, comes closest in New York to the National Health Services but is reported as serving only 5% of the New York elderly (see Table 4-1).

The New York elderly report a higher rate (14%) of hospital admissions during the previous year than do the Londoners (8%). This difference in use of medical services shows up also with respect to special medical investigations (including laboratory tests) received during the previous year. They are all more commonly reported in New York than in London. Certain fairly expensive procedures are used routinely in New York but sparingly in London.

In keeping with the greater use of medical services in New York than in London, more Londoners than New Yorkers have failed to see a doctor in the past year (25% to 17% respectively). Furthermore, more Londoners than New Yorkers have obtained prescriptions for medicine without seeing the doctor face-to-face (22% to 8% respectively). However, paradoxically, many more elderly in New York than in London claim they do not have a doctor (18% to .5% respectively). A variety of reasons are given by the New Yorkers to explain not having a doctor. Apparently many Londoners continue to identify a doctor they can turn to if needed even though they do not actually see that doctor regularly, whereas New Yorkers appear to require regular contact with their doctor in order to maintain a sense of identification.

In other ways also, the Londoners appear to feel more firmly established under the medical aegis of a doctor than do New Yorkers despite the greater medical activity that the latter experience. Forty percent of New Yorkers report there is not a doctor available to make a house call if needed in an emergency, compared to only 6% of Londoners who make this complaint.

In the same vein, Londoners much more often (94%) than New Yorkers (76%) stated that they obtain medical care through their local doctor, whereas the New Yorkers more often go to a clinic (17% vs. .3%) or outpatient department of a hospital (25% vs. 4%). Londoners (67%) see general practitioners more often than New Yorkers (59%), who see eye and ear specialists (19% vs. 4%) more often than do Londoners.

In contrast to the greater use of medical services in New York than in London, usage of non-medical practitioners (osteopaths), and podiatrists or physiotherapists is higher in London than in New York. Foot specialists (podiatrists or chiropodists) have been seen in the past month in 12% of the subjects in London and 7% in New York. The provision of foot care by a clinic is twice as common in London (21%) as in New York (10%).

As reported by subjects, cross-national differences in use of non-psychotropic medications are generally consistent with the corresponding differences in self-reports of specific physical problems. Medications for hypertension and diabetes are more commonly taken in New York than in London; the converse is true for medications for chest conditions and arthritis. However, depsite an absence of cross-national differences in affective (depressive) symptoms, Londoners report use of drugs for insomnia, barbiturates and other sedatives more often than do New Yorkers.

Medications were inventoried by the interviewer if the subject reported taking any during the past month. Subjects were asked to produce the bottles and packets of medications they were currently taking. This more objective view of medication usage was in the same direction as the cross-national differences based on self-report, though there are discrepancies in detail (104).

The greater use in New York than in London of cardiovascular medications (e.g., digitalis, cardiac glycosides, beta-adrenergic blockers, anti-arrythmics, vasodilators, etc.), antihypertensive agents (other than diuretics), and oral hypoglycemic agents or insulin, seems consistent with the respective levels of intensive medical investigations received by the elderly in the two cities. More investigations seem likely to lead to a greater rate of discovery and treatment of cardiac, hypertensive and diabetic conditions.

Psychotropic medications such as benzodiazepines (12% both cities) or barbiturates (5% both cities) are observed to be included in the stock of medications in equal frequency in the two cities, while fewer New Yorkers than Londoners took phenothiazines (0% vs. 2%) and tricyclic antidepressants or mono-amine-oxidase inhibitors (0% vs. 2%). These differences in use of psychotropics are not as marked as the subjective reports suggested.

It is difficult to relate the much higher use of vitamins in New York (15%) than in London (4%) to corresponding differences in nutritional status; presumably it reflects attitudes to preventive health practices. On the other hand, it is surprising that the frequency of the use of laxatives was equal on the two sides since one might have expected cultural attitudes to affect these rates.

B.   Formal and Informal Social Services

The personal care and support services which enable the frail and dependent elderly person, who is at risk for admission to an institution, to remain in the community include the provision of services for meals, shopping, foot care, bathing, housework and laundry, for financial supplementation and for readily available emergency help.

Table 4-6 shows that a higher proportion of the London than the New York elderly have their meals prepared for them by a formal social service. Meals-on-wheels and luncheon clubs predominate as sources of meals in London (6%) as compared with New York (.2%); however, it is worth noting that there is a counterbalancing greater use of commercial restaurants in New York (10% vs. 3%); if this is included in the reckoning then the total use of outside sources for meals is about the same in the two cities (11% in New York and 9% in London).

The use of formal social services for shopping is greater in London than in New York (5% to 1%) as it is for help with the housework (London, 10%, New York, 2%).

Some aspects of the care of the elderly are unpredictable and for this reason particularly difficult for the health and social services to manage. An example is when the elderly person is suddenly stricken and has to make emergency contact with others in order to summon help. The methods suggested for summoning help vary from using the telephone (which, as expected, is mentioned by more New Yorkers than Londoners since the latter have less access to telephones) to shouting for a neighbor, which is relied upon by nearly three times as many Londoners as New Yorkers. Two percent of the Londoners would put a card in the window to attract the attention of a passerby, but no New Yorker would rely upon that method of summoning help. The ultimate effect is that more than twice as many Londoners as New Yorkers believe they might remain unnoticed for 24 hours if they were too ill to summon help.

The social services given for personal care and support can be seen against the background of social services of a more general nature. New Yorkers find it more difficult to make ends meet than do the Londoners. Yet the Londoners are better off in terms of financial help from formal social services. Nevertheless, New Yorkers receive more help with their finances than do the Londoners because of support from children.

C.   Health Habits

Cross-national variation in habits of smoking and diet is of special interest because these habits are well known to have an influence on morbidity and mortality and can be altered by the personal resolve of the individual person.

Londoners admit to cigarette smoking more frequently (38% to 25%) than do New Yorkers, and to heavy smoking at that. This may be part of the explanation for the Londoners' higher rate of chest conditions relative to New Yorkers. Over three times as many New Yorkers as Londoners (34% vs.

10%) report being on a diet, particularly salt-free (for heart disease or hypertension), sugar-free (for diabetes), and fat-free (for weight, gall bladder problems, arteriosclerosis, etc.). The majority of those on a diet have been instructed to diet by their doctor (Table 4-7).

New Yorkers appear to be playing a more active role in controlling their own health problems than are the Londoners.

D.   Dissatisfactions Related To Service Utilization

Dissatisfactions with doctors predominate in New York (Table 4-8) although, surprisingly, dissatisfaction with costs is not a major cross-national difference. Difficulties in getting to see the doctor because of public transport problems are more common in London than in New York.

Although the depression scale as a whole showed no important cross-national differences, the items on "worry" all predominate in New York, with one of the main targets of the worrying being health (own health, other's health, other health-related problems). It is possible that the elderly living under the national health system of London have less cause to be worried by health care. It is true that Londoners are dissatisfied with the help they get from hearing aids (and other specific services) more often than New Yorkers, but presumably because the former receive hearing aids (and similar services) more often than do the latter.

The family members of the elderly person who is ill are also important targets of the health and social services. More New Yorkers than Londoners claim that a family member has a chronic illness and the various types of family stress caused by the ill family member are reported also more frequently by New Yorkers. The excess family burden in New York may be related to an excess prevalence of severely disabled or ill family members compared with London but possibly it is also related to the lesser degree to which formal social service systems intervene in New York compared with London.

E.   Supportiveness of Services

We have seen that Londoners are more likely than New Yorkers to be identified with a physician, to be able to call upon him when in need rather than go to a hospital or a clinic, to be treated at home rather than in a hospital, to receive a house call if appropriate, to be less concerned about their health, and to be satisfied with the medical service they get. In short, the Londoners appear to perceive their medical care as being more reliable and supportive. Possibly as a result, Londoners put off potential visits to their doctor more than do New Yorkers, partly, they state, because they don't want to bother the doctor (Table 4-9).

2.   COMPARISON OF SERVICES USED BY THE ELDERLY WITH
      PERVASIVE DEMENTIA OR PERVASIVE DEPRESSION

      It should be noted that the numbers of subjects in these diagnostic subgroups is small and the intergroup comparisons must therefore be viewed with caution. In the section that follows on personal time dependency, the numbers in the dependent category are larger and comparisons can be made more confidently. We have therefore chosen to present further data on formal and informal social support services in the section on dependency and not in this section on dementia and depression. Services to the dependent elderly will, of course, have relevance to dementia and depression since about 44% in New York and 19% in London of the severely dependent (warranting nursing home level of care) are demented and rates of depression are also high in those who are dependent (Table 4-10).

      The data presented in this section is thus mainly concentrated on medical services. Because of the small size of some of the groups involved we emphasize the need for caution in interpreting the comparative data and for emphasizing broad trends rather than specific findings.

      The cross-national differences in medical service utilization already reported for the cross-section of the elderly populations in the two cities are largely reflected in the services utilized by the pervasively demented and the pervasively depressed, with few qualifications (Table 4-11).

      However, an informative elaboration on the cross-section data can now be made with respect to treatment of depression: specific antidepressive medication is given to few of the pervasively depressed but more often in London than in New York; conversely, the pervasively depressed in New York receive benzodiazepines (minor tranquilizers) more often than do the Londoners. It appears that specific treatment of depression occurs more commonly in London and non-specific treatment more commonly in New York. The more ready availability of antidepressive medication in London than in New York is evident also in that two out of nine pervasively demented in London received antidepressives but none in New York.

      In certain respects, the patterns of service utilization distinguish pervasive dementia and pervasive depression from each other and the remainder of the elderly population but yet are cross-nationally consistent. In both cities, the pervasively demented are particularly likely to fail to see a doctor but be admitted to a hospital or nursing home, during the preceding year; that is, they have a tendency to receive medical services only when in dire need. Probably because of their low level of medical contact they are seldom given psychotropic medications; they are not heavily tranquilized. On the other hand, they are rarely faced with the prospect of being left to lie without help in a crisis; a reflection of the strong support network required to keep these subjects in the community (none in either city reported that they might be left alone in a crisis for 24 hours or more).

The pervasively depressed in both cities are the highest users of special investigations and are admitted to hospitals or nursing homes more often than the non-psychiatrically impaired population. As expected, they are the most likely to receive psychotropic medications. Also, more often than the other groups, the pervasively depressed believe they might, in a crisis, be left unnoticed for 24 hours or more (9% in New York and 22% in London versus 3% in New York and 11% in London of those who were neither pervasively depressed nor demented).

These data suggest that the medical service utilization patterns of these major psychiatric conditions are determined to some extent by the general tendencies of the medical systems in the two cities. Nevertheless, the distinctive natures of pervasive dementia and pervasive depression are sufficiently strong to lead to each condition having a service utilization pattern that is cross-nationally similar in important respects.

3.   COMPARISON OF SOURCES AND INTENSITY OF FORMAL AND INFORMAL SUPPORT SERVICES FOR DEPENDENT ELDERLY

It is inherent in the definition of personal time dependency, as previously given, that the group of subjects with this state will be heavy users of both formal (e.g., social agency) and informal (e.g., family) support services. Support services include those which are described in the definition of personal time dependency.

For each subject, a systematic inventory was made of the presence of primary and other providers (i.e., supporters), if any, and their professional or family affiliation, mode of reimbursement for the service provided and the frequency and duration of services. The primary provider (or supporter) is defined as the one who gives the service judged most critical to maintaining the subject at home; other ranks of providers are defined in terms of their decreasing importance in the above respect. Wherever it was difficult to judge who was the primary and who was the secondary or lower order provider, the primary label was given to the provider who contributed the most time, failing that to the provider who was a formal service agent, and failing all else to the provider who was the closest relative. Similarly, rules were constructed to resolve other difficult decisions.

Table 4-12 shows the formal and informal sources of support services given to the personal time dependent (PTD) elderly in New York and London.

Informal supporters, especially daughters, are more actively engaged in the support of the elderly in New York than in London for almost every rank of the order of providers; friends, as providers, are the exception to this cross-national trend, being more active in London than in New York.

Formal supporters are, in contrast to the informal kind, more active in London than in New York though this overall effect arises entirely from the use of public services; privately paid services are more commonly employed in New York than in London. These findings are true for almost every rank of the order of providers.

Restriction of the focus (for the sake of clarity) to primary providers reveals that informal supporters (spouse, daughter, other family and friends) are active in 80% of PTDs in New York and only 69% in London, an 11% discrepancy in favor of New York. Formal supporters as primary providers are, however, active in 22% of London PTDs and only 15% of New York cases, a discrepancy of 7% in favor of London. The corresponding cross-national contrasts are found for secondary and tertiary order providers.

In both countries informal supporters constitute the bulk of the support system for the PTD elderly but formal service in London, mostly from public agencies, are more prominent than in New York.

Table 4-13 shows the levels (intensity) of support services, formal and informal combined, given to various grades of severity of PTD of the elderly in the two cities. Levels of support are graded in terms of the institutional equivalents; that is, the formal service that would usually deliver that level of support were there no informal assistance available (see Table 4-14 for details). The severity of the PTD was based on a global rating. In both cities, the great majority of PTDs of minor severity receive the equivalent of limited home care, of moderate severity receive the equivalent of adult home care, and of marked severity receive the equivalent of nursing home care. There are, however, more of the markedly severe cases of dependency in New York than in London and there is correspondingly more nursing home equivalent care given to the community based elderly in the former than in the latter city. It should be noted that most of this nursing home equivalent care of the primary care provider is given by family members (71% in New York and 70% in London).

Tables 4-15 and 4-16 show the support services in the two cities described in terms of the level of skill and the amount of time involved on the part of the provider of formal or informal services (see Table 4-17 for guidelines to ratings). For the purposes of simplifying the cross-national comparison of skill and time involved in support services, a single index has been calculated in the form of the hypothetical cost of these services were the prevailing labor costs in New York to be applied to the services in both cities. This cost, given in dollars, summarizes in a standard manner the effort resulting from the skill and time of the provider irrespective of the actual amount and source of payment; it is shown in Table 4-18. Approximately the same total amount of effort is expended in both cities but the distribution of the effort is different; in New York most of the effort goes into full-time or daily personal care while in London it goes into daily or half-daily housekeeping. That finding is consistent with there being, as suggested above, more severely dependent elderly persons in the community in New York than in London; it also underlines the different structuring of the support system in the two cities in terms of levels of service.

Table 4-19 shows the level of support services given to the elderly in the two cities with respect to the effect of increasing age. In both cities the lesser levels of care are given mainly to the 'young-old' age groups. However, in New York a greater proportion of every age group than in London receives the most intensive type of home care (i.e., comparable to a nursing home).

Table 4-1. Use of Third Party Payments by the Elderly in
New York and London*

Item Content	New York %	London %
Subject covered by National Health Service	0	96
Subject covered by Medicaid	17	0
Subject covered by Medicare A	91	0
Subject covered by Medicare B	83	0
Subject covered by Blue Cross	25	0
Subject covered by Blue Shield	31	0
Subject covered by HIP	5	0
Subject covered by other health insurance	9	1

*The chi square was used to compare percents with problems in
New York City and London by testing for significant differences.
Only items showing statistically significant differences at the
.05 level are included in this table.

Table 4-2. Use of Medical Services by the Elderly in
New York and London*

Item Content	New York %	London %
Was in hospital or nursing home during past year	14	8
In past year had chest x-ray	60	25
In past year had blood test	70	30
In past year had urine test	71	26
In past year had ECG	63	16
In past year had blood pressure test	82	47
In past year had rectal exam	41	11

*The chi square was used to compare percents with problems in
New York City and London by testing for significant differences.
Only items showing statistically significant differences at the
.05 level are included in this table.

Table 4-3.   Contacts with Medical Practitioners by the Elderly in New York and London

Item Content	New York %	London %
Does not have a doctor	18	0.5
Has a doctor but:		
can't give doctor's name	6	0.6
If doesn't have doctor, why?		
doesn't have doctor because doctor died	2	0
doesn't have doctor because doesn't need one	6	0
doesn't have own doctor because uses clinic	6	0
doesn't see doctor because is scornful of them	2	0
has other reason for not having doctor	3	0.3
Claims not having doctor is a problem	2	0.3
Has seen a doctor in past year	83	75
Has obtained prescription without seeing doctor	8	22

(continues)

Table 4-3. continued

Item Content	New York %	London %
Has seen general practitioner in last year	59	67
Has seen eye/ear specialist	19	4
Has seen foot specialist in past month	7	12
Foot clinic helps with foot care	10	21
Lack of public transport leads to difficulties in seeing doctor	1	4
No doctor will make a house call	40	6
Goes to local doctor for medical care	76	94
Goes to clinic for medical care	17	0.3
Goes to out-patient hospital department for medical care	25	4
Other source of medical care	8	1

*The chi square was used to compare percents with problems in New York City and London by testing for significant differences. Only items showing statistically significant differences at the .05 level are included in this table.

Table 4-4. Self-report of Drug Use by the Elderly in
New York and London*

Item Content	New York %	London %
Non-psychotropic drugs		
Takes pain killer	20	13
Takes blood pressure drug	24	13
Takes drug for chest condition	3	10
Takes diabetes drug	8	3
Takes arthritis drug	10	15
Psychotropic drugs		
Takes drug for insomnia	8	14
Takes barbiturates	2	5
Takes other sedatives	2	8

*The chi square was used to compare percents with problems in
New York City and London by testing for significant differences.
Only items showing statistically significant differences at the
.05 level are included in this table.

Table 4-5. Generic Medications Identified by Interviewer
in New York and London (Not Restricted to
Cross-Nationally Significant Differences)

Item Content	New York %	London %
Blood pressure medication other than diuretic	11	7
Diuretic	11	15
Antiarrhythmias	2	0
Vasodilators	5	4
Other cardiac medications	2	0.3
Anti-inflammatory agents	3	9
Systemic corticosteroids	3	1
Aspirin	5	2
Non-aspirin analgesics	6	12
Narcotics and codeine	3	0.5
Oral hypoglycemics	6	2
Insulin	1	0
Bronchodilators and asthma remedies	2	5
Cough and cold remedies	2	2
Antihistamines	1	2
Vitamins	15	4
Laxatives	8	8
Psychotropic		
Antidepressants (tricyclics or MAO inhibitors)	0	2
Benzodiazepines	12	12
Barbiturates	5	5
Phenothiazines	0	2

Table 4-6. Personal Care and Support Services of the Elderly in New York and London*

I tem Content	New York %	London %
Assistance with Activities of Daily Living		
someone else prepares meals for subject	20	32
receives meals on wheels	0	2
has regular meals at commercial eating establishment	10	3
has regular meal at luncheon club	.2	4
uses social service for help with shopping	1	5
does own shopping but with help	7	2
gets help with bathing	1	3
difficulty getting help with housework due to reluctance or lack of initiative	0	2
living companion helps with housework	4	.5
social agency helps with housework	2	10
maid helps with housework	2	.5
other helps with housework	4	.5
family member outside household helps with laundry	2	4
other person helps with laundry	3	.5

(continues)

Table 4-6. continued

Item Content	New York %	London %
Summoning Help		
does not have a phone	7	41
no access to telephone	3	16
does not mention a plausible means of summoning help which is immediately accessible	15	31
would use own phone to summon help	56	36
would use other phone to summon help	2	8
gives public emergency phone number	28	3
gives personal phone number and back up	23	7
would put card in window to get help	0	2
would shout to attract neighbor	9	25
would use some other method to get help	6	2
might go 24 hours without help	6	14

(continues)

Table **4-6.** continued

Item Content	New York %	London %
Financial Support		
money tight	27	9
subject admits to financial problem	19	7
has trouble paying for food	7	2
has trouble paying for rent	10	2
has trouble paying for utilities	2	0.5
rater finds subject has financial problem	19	5
subject has financial problem but receives no social service aid	7	2
subject is receiving financial aid but not enough	10	1
children give money	15	4
other relatives give money	2	0.3
has a bus pass	63	73
receives food stamps	1	7
receives tax rebate for property	4	9
receives rent rebate	8	20

*The chi square was used to compare percents with problems in New York City and London by testing for significant differences. Only items showing statistically significant differences at the .05 level are included in this table.

Table 4-7.   Health Habits of the Elderly in New York
             and London*

Item Content	New York %	London %
Has smoked during past month	25	38
Has smoked 10 or more cigarettes daily	20	38
On a diet	34	10
Type of diet:		
Salt-free diet	18	1
Sugar-free diet	12	3
Fat-free diet	8	2
Avoids certain other foods	11	6
Diet medically prescribed	25	9
Self-imposed diet	4	2
Diet to control heart disease	11	1
Other purpose of diet	10	2

*The chi square was used to compare percents with problems in New York City and London by testing for significant differences. Only items showing statistically significant differences at the .05 level are included in this table.

Table 4-8.   Satisfaction with Services by the Elderly in
             New York and London*

I tem Content	New York %	London %
Dissatisfied with health care		
Dissatisfied with doctor's treatment	14	7
Cost of medical care led to dissatisfaction	2	0
Other reason for dissatisfaction	3	1
Worries		
Worrying bothersome	26	15
Worries about own health	20	15
Worries about others' health	19	12
Worries about other health related problems	8	2
Worries over finances	12	7
Worries about inflation	3	0
Looks worried	16	7
Dissatisfied with hearing aid		
Hearing aid doesn't improve hearing	2	5
Inadequate aid is reason for turning aid off	0.2	5
Discomfort with hearing aid	1	3
Leaves aid off because of cosmetic reasons	1	4
Difficulty with hearing interferes with things would like to do	5	13

(continues)

Table 4-8. continued

Item Content	New York %	London %
Family burden		
Family member has chronic physical sickness	9	4
Family member has memory loss	3	1
Dependent family member causes financial strain	4	1
Has affected health	5	2
Interferes with sleep	7	3

*The chi square was used to compare percents with problems in New York City and London by testing for significant differences. Only items showing statistically significant differences at the .05 level are included in this table.

Table 4-9.   Seeking Medical Care by the Elderly in New York and London*

Item Content	New York %	London %
Puts off seeking medical care	21	29
Puts off seeking medical care because too costly	2	0
Puts off seeking medical care because doesn't want to bother doctor	1	13

*The chi square was used to compare percents with problems in New York City and London by testing for significant differences. Only items showing statistically significant differences at the .05 level are included in this table.

Table 4-10.   Pervasively Demented or Depressed by Personal Time Dependency in New York and London

	New York City %	New York City N	London %	London N
Pervasively demented and PTD (nursing home level of care)	44	(19)	19	(5)
Pervasively depressed and PTD (all levels of care)	16	(21)	19	(23)

Table 4-11. Percentage of Elderly with Pervasive Dementia or Pervasive Depression Using Medical Services in New York and London

	Pervasively Demented		Pervasively Depressed		Neither	
	New York N=22 %	London N=9 %	New York N=58 %	London N=49 %	New York N=365 %	London N=338 %
MEDICAL ATTENTION						
Does not have doctor	30	0	7	2	19	1
Has not seen or consulted doctor in past year	16	33	7	18	19	26
Special Investigations:						
Chest x-ray	75	25	73	29	57	21
Blood test	77	25	84	39	67	25
Urine	88	38	78	27	69	22
EKG	77	13	73	18	60	13
Blood pressure	88	38	91	41	78	41
Inpatient Treatment:						
In hospital/nursing home						
over past year	25	22	18	19	12	7
Week or less	5	0	4	0	3	1
Week to a month	15	11	11	6	7	3
More than a month	5	11	4	13	2	3
Psychotropic:* (identified by interviewer)						
Antidepressants	0	22	3	14	0	0
Benzodiazepines	5	11	31	18	6	10
Barbiturates	5	0	3	6	1	3
Phenothiazines	5	0	2	2	0	0
Other	5	22	3	16	3	10

*A random subsample (New York, N=70 and London, N=72) was used for the calculation of numbers and percentages for use of psychotropic medications by the elderly who were neither pervasively depressed nor pervasively demented.

Table 4-12. Formal and Informal Support Services for the Personal Time Dependent Elderly in New York and London

Order of Provider

Type of Provider	Primary		Secondary		Tertiary		Quarternary		Total Providers	
	New York N=132	London N=124	New York N=71	London N=53	New York N=27	London N=24	New York N=4	London N=8	New York N=234	London N=209
Spouse	29%	30%	6%	-	7%	-	-	-	19%	18%
Daughter	34%	22%	25%	11%	11%	8%	25%	12%	29%	17%
Other Family	14%	11%	35%	23%	30%	25%	25%	25%	22%	16%
Friend	3%	6%	14%	19%	22%	25%	25%	38%	9%	12%
Private Nurse	-	1%	3%	-	4%	-	-	-	1%	0.5%
Private Aide	3%	-	-	-	-	-	-	-	2%	-
Private Home Helper	5%	5%	7%	-	7%	4%	-	-	6%	3%
Public Nurse	1%	2%	-	8%	-	8%	-	-	1%	4%
Public Aide	1%	2%	1%	-	-	-	-	-	1%	1%
Public Home Helper	5%	12%	3%	24%	-	8%	-	12%	4%	15%
Other*	5%	9%	6%	15%	19%	21%	25%	12%	7%	12%
TOTAL	100%	100%	100%	100%	100%	100%	100%	100%	100%	100%

Note: In some cases percents do not total exactly 100% due to rounding errors.

*Includes transportation services, meals on wheels, day care centers, etc.

Table 4-13. The Level of Support Services Given to the Personal Time Dependent Elderly in New York and London

Institutional Equivalent of Support Service*	Severity of Personal Time Dependency															
	Minor				Moderate				Marked				Total			
	New York		London		New York		London		New York		London		New York		London	
		N		N		N		N		N		N		N		N
Limited Home Care	23%	(31)	31%	(39)	9%	(11)	6%	(7)	2%	(2)	1%	(1)	34%	(44)	38%	(47)
Adult Home	5%	(7)	3%	(4)	24%	(30)	35%	(44)	5%	(8)	2%	(2)	34%	(45)	40%	(50)
Nursing Home	0%	(0)	1%	(1)	2%	(2)	6%	(7)	30%	(41)	15%	(19)	32%	(43)	22%	(27)
Total	28%	(38)	35%	(44)	35%	(43)	47%	(58)	37%	(51)	18%	(22)	100%	(132)	100%	(124)

*refer to text.

Table 4-14. Definitions of Level of Support Services to
Community Residents Viewed as the Equivalent
of Institutional Services (where required
for a disability)

EQUIVALENT TO LIMITED HOME CARE:

Any one of either:

Shopping, cooking or housekeeping.

EQUIVALENT TO ADULT HOME:

Any two of the following:

Shopping, cooking, housekeeping; or special accommodation or
relocation to provide elevators or single level stairs;
frequent administrative or semi-legal advice; constant
company, security or encouragement; heavy chores.

EQUIVALENT TO HEALTH-RELATED FACILITY OR
SKILLED NURSING FACILITY:

Qualifies for Adult Home and any one of following:

Supervision with bathing, walking, grooming and medications;
changing bandages, care of incision, immediate response to
falls or confusion; assistance with dressing, grooming,
bathing, walking, shifting in bed, feeding, standing, care of
incontinence, prevention of wandering or dangerous behavior,
rehabilitation, observation for those who cannot communicate
or are not aware of needs; includes individuals who require
round-the-clock nursing services.

Table 4-15. Comparison of Level of Skill Performed by Primary Providers of Support to Personal Time Dependent Elderly in New York and London

		PRIMARY PROVIDERS		
Level of Skill Performed*		New York		London
Nursing	2	2%	4	3%
Personal Care	45	34%	18	15%
Housekeeping	49	37%	86	69%
Admin/Errands	31	23%	11	9%
Company	5	4%	5	4%
Total	132	100%	124	100%

*For definitions, refer to Table 4-17.

Table 4-16. Comparison of Time Spent by Primary Providers of Support to Personal Time Dependent Elderly in New York and London

		PRIMARY PROVIDERS		
Time Spent by Primary Provider for PTD*		New York		London
Full Time	16	12%	13	11%
Daily	32	24%	16	13%
Half Days	25	19%	40	32%
Short Sessions	41	31%	44	36%
Weekly	18	14%	11	8%
Total	132	100%	124	100%

*For definitions, refer to Table 4-17.

Table 4-17.　Levels of Skill and Time Commitment of Provider

Level of Time Commitment		Level of Skill*				
Hours Per Week		Skilled	Personal	House-keeping	Admin./ Errands	Compan-ionship
Full time or live in	80 hrs					
Daily (working day)	40 hrs					
Half days**	16 hrs					
Short sessions**	8 hrs					
Weekly	4 hrs					
Monthly or less	2 hrs					

*Levels of Skill

Skilled care:　Nursing of wounds, medical house-calls, care of catheter, etc.

Personal care:　Dressing, shifting in bed, transferring, bathing, feeding, assisting, walking, care of incontinence, prevention of exposure to common danger, prevention of wandering, anticipation of basic needs if not communicated, grooming, supervision of medication, etc.

Housekeeping:　Cooking, cleaning, mending, heavy chores, preparing food, etc.

Admin./
Errands:　Shopping, planning, budgeting, procuring devices, arranging relocation, etc.

Companionship:　Reassurance, company, encouragement to maintain at least minimal activities and interest, escort on excursions, being responsive to emergencies such as falls or fits.

**Individuals receiving full-time services, but only infrequently (say 4-8 weeks a year) are placed in these categories if seen in an interval status. In all other cases the status over the past month is judged.

Table 4-18. The Costs (in Dollars) of the Support System: Primary Providers Only for New York and London

Levels of Skill

Times per week	Nursing		Personal Care		Housekeeping		Administration/ Errands		Company		Total	
	N.Y.	London	N.Y.	London	N.Y.	London	N.Y.	London	N.Y.	London	N.Y.	London
Full	286	286	1849	713	143	715	–	–	–	254	2278	1968
Daily	–	–	3329	432	1170	1430	–	–	–	212	4499	2074
Half-daily	–	–	232	348	988	1768	43	–	54	–	1317	2116
Short sess.	–	31	116	58	364	832	423	190	81	–	984	1111
Weekly	–	16	14	28	18	39	106	21	13	13	152	117
Total	286	333	5540	1579	2683	4784	572	211	148	479	9229	7386

*Based on figures from State of New York, Department of Labor, Division of Research and Statistics, Wage Report No. 255, October 1977.

Table 4-19. The Relationship Between Age and Institutional
Equivalents of Service to the Personal Time
Dependent Elderly in New York and London

New York

AGE OF PTD'S	INSTITUTIONAL EQUIVALENTS OF SERVICE			TOTAL (N=132)	
	LIMITED HOME CARE	ADULT HOME	NURSING HOME		
65 - 69	46%	29%	25%	100%	(N=24)
70 - 74	48%	21%	31%	100%	(N=29)
75 - 79	25%	47%	28%	100%	(N=32)
80 +	22%	33%	43%	100%	(N=46)
Unknown (N=1)					

x^2 = 80.4, d.f.=6
Significance $p = \leq 0.001$

London

AGE OF PTD'S	INSTITUTIONAL EQUIVALENTS OF SERVICE			TOTAL (N=124)	
	LIMITED HOME CARE	ADULT HOME	NURSING HOME		
65 - 69	57%	26%	17%	100%	(N=23)
70 - 74	42%	33%	25%	100%	(N=24)
75 - 79	40%	49%	11%	100%	(N=35)
80 +	24%	45%	31%	100%	(N=42)

x^2 = 61.6, d.f.=6
Significance $p = \leq 0.01$

Section V
Conclusion

The preceding pages have been heavily weighted with the presentation of method and data. Relatively little space has been given to inferences which attempt to relate the findings to the aims of this study; namely, to compare cross-nationally between New York and London the frequency, form and associations of psychiatric conditions in the community elderly with a view to furthering understanding of the nature and care of mental disorder in old age. This concluding chapter is an opportunity to draw together the major findings of this study and show their application to understanding the nature and care of three key health problems of psychiatric relevance in old age: dementia, depression, and disability. The latter condition, while not a conventional psychiatric category, stands so often in a causal or consequential relation to psychiatric disorder that it has great psychiatric relevance.

The conclusions in this chapter will reflect not only the data so far presented but also supporting data from other United States-United Kingdom Cross-National Project studies which were later carried out between 1977-81. The U.S.-U.K. series of studies began in 1966 and are ongoing; they are linked to each other by method, cross-national geography and a mental health theme which makes for interrelated findings; furthermore, from 1972 onwards the studies have focused on the geriatric age range.

Citations are provided in this chapter for the details of data or analyses which are discussed but not fully presented here. The subject matter of the citations falls into the following groups:

(1) Further analyses of data from initial interviews in the U.S.-U.K. Geriatric Community Study (5-11, 14).

(2) Data from a one-year follow-up of the U.S.-U.K. Geriatric Community Study subjects in New York and London. Rates of mortality and institutional admission were determined for the whole sample and diagnostic groups in each city, and the CARE interview was repeated whenever the

subject was available and cooperative: 292 subjects in New York and 224 in London (20).

(3) A longitudinal study of a subset (N=110) of the geriatric community sample in New York, who had been interviewed in an independent study five years previous to the Geriatric Community Study (9).

(4) A study of a representative sample of the elderly in long term care facilities in New York (N=162) and London (N=159) (25). This study was designed as the complement of the Community Study so that together the two studies would come close to representing the universe of elderly in the two cities.

(5) A comparison of the treatment and outcome of matched groups of frail elderly in institutions and alternative care settings in New York and London (37-39).

The U.S.-U.K. Geriatric Community Study produced not only substantive findings but also a method for cross-national geriatric studies and, equally useful, a systematic assessment technique for comprehensive evaluation of the health and social problems of old age. This chapter will include a review of these methodological contributions of the U.S.-U.K. Project and will provide a summary of developments in the U.S.-U.K. assessment techniques between 1977-1981.

This monograph is a report on the work of the U.S.-U.K. Project. Thus, the conclusions are largely restricted to U.S.-U.K. Project data or papers written by Project staff. This limitation of scope is determined by reasons of space and emphasis and is not an oversight of the importance of the work of other investigators in the field of the epidemiology of geriatric mental health or in the cross-national arena, which has been properly acknowledged in other publications by U.S.-U.K. Project members.

1.   ADVANCES IN METHOD

The U.S.-U.K. Cross-National Project has demonstrated by its longevity and productivity that its organization and methods are effective means of conducting cross-national studies. During the Project's fifteen year history of continuity in research work it has completed five major cross-national studies (Adult Diagnostic Project, Psychogeriatric Hospital Study, Geriatric Community Study, Geriatric Institutional Study, Alternatives to Institutional Care Study) and is now embarked on a sixth (Geriatric Mental Health Problems in Primary Care). The Project staff have published more than 100 papers, chapters or books based on the data, methods or concepts originating in this series of studies. The management of this endeavour has a bearing on the potential for development of successful and enduring collaborative work in geriatric mental health both within and between countries. The assessment techniques resulting from the U.S.-U.K. series have also a wide application outside of the cross-national context.

The organizational strength of the U.S.-U.K. Project springs from a collaboration between two teams with equal standing, one in New York and the other in London (1, 13). Whatever the source of funding, neither of the two teams dominates the other. The aims and methods of each study are decided jointly and unanimously. Each team, being cognizant of local conditions can ensure that the aims have significance for each country and that the methods are as culture-fair as possible. Each side is responsible for local data collection but training is carried out together and there are frequent exchanges of personnel. Structured interview techniques and accompanying training manuals operationalize methods sufficiently to achieve and maintain internationally reliable assessment. Both sides have equal access to data and credit for publication is shared between the teams. These principles are designed to maintain a bond of trust between the two sides. Trust is crucial to weathering the stresses that confront the Project, typically at the following junctures:

(1) When the detailed content for the structured interviews is debated. Since the content of the interview will become a persistent influence on the interviewer for a lengthy period of time and will constrain the hypotheses that can be tested, its details are likely to be taken very seriously.

(2) When individual team members develop personal research agendas which are tangential to the overall aims of the Project.

(3) When data collection reaches its later and usually more difficult stages; that is, when recalcitrant and hard-to-reach subjects are approached.

(4) When deadline pressures mount for exchanges of drafts of publications.

The stability of the collaborating arrangement over the years not only fosters trust between team members but also aids the adoption of a method of interview by creating a traditional style of assessment within the Project teams, allows new studies to be planned while conducting an existing study, and permits continuing analyses of previous and aggregated studies.

The traditional style of assessment for health and social problems, as built up in the U.S.-U.K. Project, is based on semi-structured interviewing techniques and tailored to the special characteristics of the elderly subject (3, 52, 54). The experience of the U.S.-U.K. Project is that the vast majority of the community elderly will accept a lengthy interview, even longer than 1-1/2 hours, provided that the interview is understandable, meaningful, tactful, and has a measured pace. The central assessment instrument used in the U.S.-U.K. Geriatric Community Study is the Comprehensive Assessment and Referral Evaluation (CARE) (4). In order to make this approach understandable to the subject the questions are made as concise and straightforward as possible; questions with multiple qualifiers or clauses, which are not quickly grasped by many elderly, are presented as several separate questions. The clustering of topics in the CARE is arranged in a way that is logical to the subject, not according to professional logic; for example, problems with sleep are covered in a sequence rather than being fragmented into sections dealing with the various causes of sleep disturbance such as depression, physical disorder, or social disruptions. The meaningfulness of the interview is enhanced by its scope which includes a sufficiently wide range of problems (and assets) as to allow the subject to describe a substantial part of their daily concerns and interests. However, there is enough flexibility in the administration of the interview to let the interviewer follow the subject's lead in selecting the order in which topics are discussed. In order to reduce stress on the subject, the questions dealing with psychiatric disorder are dispersed in the instrument among questions dealing with related but non-psychiatric problems; for example, physical and social impediments to going out alone are juxtaposed with questions on anxiety of the agoraphobic (fear of open spaces) type. Thus, the subject is protected from feeling that the interviewer is persevering in trying to unearth evidence of psychiatric disorder, a matter about which many elderly are sensitive. In the same vein, tests of intellectual performance are presented either at the beginning of the interview where they can be seen as gathering routine identifying information (age, address, etc.) or interspersed among tests of neurological function.

The reduction of stress to the subject by the steps outlined above is important for gaining acceptability of the interview and for facilitating optimal performance by the subject. Proceeding through the interview in an unhurried manner also helps to reduce tension in the subject. The orderly nature of the assessment technique guides the interviewer through consideration of numerous and complex issues with a maximum of efficiency and also a steady pace. Should it be necessary to divide the interview into more than one session the structure will assist the later consolidation of the resulting information.

Very few subjects prematurely terminated a CARE interview; yet for patients who had multiple problems, or were frail or discursive the duration of the interview was frequently over 2 hours. When the CARE was originally constructed in 1973-74 there was almost no empirical data with respect to the community elderly to guide the development of a more efficient instrument, i.e., one that would collect the minimum necessary information in the least amount of time. However, the U.S.-U.K. Geriatric Community data allowed further advances in achieving an efficient instrument (22). Four kinds of more efficient instruments have been developed from the CARE:

(1)   comprehensive but shorter such as the CORE-CARE;

(2)   targeting selected health and social problems such as the SHORT-CARE for depression, dementia, and disability (23);

(3)   adaptations for other specific settings such as the INSTIT-CARE for use in long term care facilities (25); and

(4)   the MERGE-CARE for use in primary medical, nursing or social work practice (99).

The CORE-CARE is composed of those items (scripted questions and defined responses) in the CARE which proved to be most useful in the Community Study; namely, the items which formed relatively independent homogeneous scales with high internal consistency, occurred with reasonable frequency in the general population of elderly, were not redundant to items already selected, were most discriminating between diagnostic categories, and were most sensitive to change over 1 year. Items were also retained on the basis of judgement and to maintain a smooth flow to the interview. The 1500 items in the CARE were thus reduced to 314 in the scales of the CORE-CARE. The latter instrument has been used in several surveys by U.S.-U.K. Project members and also by other investigators (105-108). The CORE-CARE data can be analyzed by key individual items, scale scores, latent class categories, diagnostic scales, and global ratings; or by diagnoses made according to the criteria developed in the Community Study and described in this report and elsewhere (10, 14).

Whereas the CARE, CORE-CARE, and INSTIT-CARE are essentially research and needs assessment instruments, the MERGE-CARE was a variant intended for case management of elderly patients in primary care settings. The topics and

items are designed to evaluate problems of relevance to
primary care (whether in a medical, nursing, or social
setting) but which often receive insufficient attention: for
examples, non-compliance with treatment, weak social
supports, environmental barriers to health-care, poor
nutrition, early warning signs of cancer, dental problems,
perceptual difficulties and health problems overshadowed by
the presenting complaint. In addition to discrete items of
information, common problems are defined and also evaluated
globally with a method for indicating action plans where
appropriate. The assessment technique can be a device to
facilitate the coordination and monitoring of a network of
services for the multi-problem patient.

A training program for interviewers of the CARE and its
variants has been constructed and its impact on improving
reliability demonstrated in a study involving the SHORT-CARE
(22). The program takes 5 days to administer to a group of
5-10 trainees, provided they have some background in the
health sciences or in systematic method. Interdisciplinary
reliability is good and the interview can be administered by
psychiatrists, physicians, nurses, psychologists, social
workers or social scientists.

The content of the CARE and some of its variants are
further discussed elsewhere (23). The original version gave
equal attention to psychiatric, medical and social problems
but later versions have a varying emphasis depending on the
purpose and setting for which it is developed.

The geriatric assessment methods of the U.S.-U.K.
Project, from the Geriatric Mental State Schedule (54) which
preceded the CARE to the currently evolving MERGE-CARE, have
been characterized by their clinical orientation. The item
content, scales, global ratings and diagnostic criteria are
directed at identifying problems that have specific
health-care implications. Thus the assessment is designed to
distinguish between clinical and non-clinical patterns of
symptoms or situations: a clinical pattern is one that would
impel a clinician of the health or social service professions
to intervene. Particular examples of this focus are the
distinction between clinical (pervasive) depression and the
normal spectrum of unhappiness, clinical (pervasive) dementia
and the normal age changes in intellectual functioning, and
clinical (personal time) dependency and the normal decline in
physical capacity with age. Similarly, items are included to
distinguish psychiatric, physical, social or normal types of
such complaints as sleep disturbance, loss of weight,
perceptual problems, breathlessness, social contacts, fear of
crime, inadequacies in housing, etc. Because of this
clinical slant, the CARE and its variants have proved useful
for studies of the nature and care of the health and social

problems of old age, for needs assessment surveys, and for case management in service settings.

2. DEMENTIA

Dementia is a term covering a variety of conditions in which there is deterioration of the mature intellect, a strong tendency to progressive decline and disability and a shortened life expectancy (41). It is to be expected that in a series of cases labelled as dementia, the majority will be of the Alzheimer type involving a primary disorder of neurones and characteristic neuropathology, a substantial minority will be due to arteriosclerotic changes which cause anoxic damage to brain tissue, and a smaller minority will be secondary to potentially reversible factors which alter physiological functioning of the brain; in addition, there will be an uncertain proportion who are not demented but are misdiagnosed as such (62). The conditions that are most commonly misdiagnosed as dementia in old age include depression, acute confusional (delirious) state, aphasias (which interfere with coherent communication) and life-long mental retardation. The frequency of misdiagnosis will largely depend on the accuracy and completeness of information collected about the subject's condition through examination, testing and informants' reports, the duration of observation, the criteria used for diagnosis, the availability of special investigations and the presence of diagnostic bias.

The indicators of dementia used in this study consisted of rational and homogeneous scales, a latent class, global ratings, and diagnosis.

(1) The content of the scales covers the key symptoms of dementia: disorientation and impairment of recent memory. However, these symptoms are shared by all of the subtypes of dementia and also by acute confusional states and some of the conditions subject to misdiagnosis as dementia. The scales therefore have the advantage of providing a score for each and every subject so that the distribution of numbers of symptoms can be compared cross-nationally, but the disadvantage of being imprecise in classifying cases. Nevertheless, high scores are very likely to indicate cases of dementia (60).

(2) Diagnoses were made clinically and also according to criteria designed for use in this study. The criterion-based diagnosis (pervasive dementia) was of good and interdisciplinary reliability and has been shown to be at least as valid as clinical diagnosis in terms of predicting outcomes consistent with the expected course of dementia (14). The criterion-based diagnosis was of particular value

to this study because it could be applied uniformly to
information irrespective of whether a psychiatrist had
interviewed the case and regardless of the city in which the
subject lived.

Whereas the scale scores are largely restricted to a
description of the subject's intellectual symptoms at a point
in time, the diagnoses took into account aspects of the
chronology and course of the symptoms, associated conditions
and alternative diagnoses such as depression. The diagnoses
could therefore be more specific than the scales to dementia
and its major subtypes, within the constraints of a single
interview of questionnaire and test format. The scale scores
and the diagnosis of pervasive dementia were the main frames
of reference for the cross-national comparison of dementia.

It was quite unexpected that rates of dementia, however
measured, were significantly higher in New York than in
London. There was no theory about the causation of dementia
that would have led us to expect this finding and there is
still no adequate explanation for it. The cross-national
differences were of the order of two-fold for scale scores,
latent classes, and diagnosis. More convincingly, the
direction of the differences was consistent for each of the
five random subsamples of elderly subjects in each city.
Taking into account the effects of age, sex, immigration,
race, education, and subtype of dementia did not wash out the
observed excess of dementia in New York.

There have been a number of independent studies which
have reported rates of dementia in various populations (45).
These rates have varied between studies, but this has
generally been explained away as a function of differing
diagnostic criteria or demographic profiles. However, the
New York-London differences reported here cannot readily be
dismissed on grounds of diagnosis or demography. Moreover,
the one year follow-up on these cases gave no reason to
believe that the initial diagnosis had been wrong: the cases
of pervasive dementia either died, were admitted to
institutions or continued to be intellectually impaired (20).
It is to be emphasized that this diagnosis referred only to
cases that were definitely demented with clearcut signs of
consequent disability in the activities of daily living. A
careful search for concomitant symptoms of depression was
always conducted and in those few cases where depression was
present as well as dementia the latter symptoms were regarded
as primary only when they clearly predominated.

The follow-up study (20) showed that the dementias in
New York had a higher mortality rate (33%) than those in
London (0%); this makes it less likely that a longer duration
of the course of dementia could account for the higher
prevalence rates in New York. The number of new cases

classified by latent class analysis as demented on reexamination at one year follow-up was higher in New York (2.4%) than in London (.4%) suggesting that incidence rates show cross-national trends in the same direction as the prevalence rates. The number of case of latent class dementia at one year follow-up was still about twice as high in New York (6.2%) as in London (3.1%). On the homogeneous scale of organic brain syndrome (dementia) the mean score at follow-up was 1.1 in New York and 0.5 in London.

Selection out of the community and into institutions could in theory account for the lower rates of dementia in London but virtually the same proportion of the London dementias (11.1%) as New York dementias (9.5%) entered institutions during the follow-up year. Moreover, the later U.S.-U.K. Project's Institutional Study (25) did not find higher rates of dementia in long-term care facilities of London than of New York, while the overall proportion of the elderly population in institutions was slightly lower in London than in New York.

It is possible that had the non-responders in each city been included 'in the assessments, then the differences in rates of dementia would have been ironed out. Compared with census data the New York sample was skewed towards females 75 and over (40% for the sample vs. 35% for the census) as opposed to those 65-74 yrs. In London the fit between census and study data was closer. However, adjusting age and sex so as to match the New York and London samples did not reduce the cross-national difference in rates of dementia. Moreover, the New York-London ratio of dementia remained in the same direction and magnitude even where response rates varied between the subsamples and also at follow-up where the response rate was higher in New York (72%) than in London (63%). In addition, the differences with respect to dementia stand out against the prevailing cross-national similarities in most other health problems.

The higher mortality rate of dementias in New York than in London during the follow-up year (20) confirms that the diagnosis of this condition was not broader or looser in New York than in London and is consistent with other evidence that at initial interview there were more severe cases in New York than in London.

Despite attempts to control many of the methodological and selective factors that could account for the cross-national differences in dementia rates, it is still not possible to rule out non-etiological factors as explanations of the differences. It remains for these findings to be replicated; prior to that it is not useful to speculate on whether true cross-national differences in the incidence or prevalence of dementia can provide clues to the etiology of

Alzheimer's, multi-infarct, or other subtypes of dementia. However, it is no longer justified to dismiss differences in rates of dementia between these two cities as a simple methodological artifact.

There were cross-national differences also, in the provision of services to the cases of dementia. They were reflective, for the most part, of non-specific differences applying to most health problems: more visits to the doctor and special investigations in New York and more home care and house calls services in London. Lack of use of general practitioners (primary medical care) was a more common occurrence for the dementias in New York. However, it was of great interest that only one case (in New York) was on a major tranquilizer (phenothiazine); a dramatic contrast with the results of the U.S.-U.K. Project's Institutional Study where in New York about 40% of the residents with dementia were on a major tranquilizer, in London, about one in five (25).

Several generalities arise from this study that apply across the two cities to cases of dementia in the community. Only a very small proportion of the community population 65 years and older could be definitely diagnosed as dementia; in the region of 2.5-5%. In the U.S.-U.K. Project's Institutional Study about 40% of the residents of long term care facilities were found to be suffering from dementia, which constitutes another 2.5% of the general elderly population (25). Combining the community and institutional samples gives a total figure of 5-7.5% of the elderly with dementia. Even in the age group over 80 years, the rates of dementia were about 20%. Nevertheless, this small proportion with dementia constitute a large proportion of the severely disabled elderly in the community (and in institutions). The extent to which dementia accounts for the dependency of old age is underlined by this study. At the same time, it is clear that the vast majority of elderly remain intellectually alert to an advanced age.

The strongest associations of dementia in this study, as determined by relationships between rational scale scores, is with age, inadequate activities, disability and mortality; the first of these associations is assumed to be a partial cause and the others, consequences of dementia. With respect to age, there is a dramatic contrast in rates of dementia between the groups younger and older than 75 years; the exception is the lack of increased dementia scores in older men in London. Although the numbers of the latter group are too small to allow emphasis of this finding, it is nonetheless of interest that this particular group of elderly men have been highly selected by war mortality and by emigration. Apart from this, there is no consistent relationship between gender and dementia scores that could not be attributed to there being more elderly women than elderly men in the population.

An intriguing inverse relationship was noted between dementia scores and level of education and occupation. This association is partly a confounding of cohort (generational) and age effects: education is increasing with successive cohorts so that it is lowest in the oldest age group whereas dementia scores are highest. Nevertheless, a relationship is still evident when age is held constant; the implications of this finding have been discussed at length elsewhere (7).

The cases of dementia identified in each city were mostly still alive, though a few were in institutions, at the one year follow-up (20). The cases of dementia in New York who were 80 years or older did not even have a higher mortality rate than did age-matched controls. The younger dementias did have an abnormally high mortality rate (20). There were no deaths among the dementias in London during the follow-up period. A strong impression is gained of the elderly with disabling dementia receiving care in the community, mostly from their families, for long periods of time. This long duration of care may provide a more difficult challenge to family and home care services than do acute time-limited conditions or terminal states. A substantial part of the life of the family member is involved and changes in their health and morale during this period of time will influence their capacity to maintain their caring role. For home care services, this long duration of need means that their case-load is likely to accumulate; furthermore, a commitment of a certain level of services to an individual may slip gradually into a higher level as the person's dementing condition deteriorates.

The data on the level of services provided by the New York and London home care services suggest that in London there is a more strict limit set to the level of home services provided; presumably the person who deteriorates beyond a point at which that level of services is adequate is likely to be transferred to an institutional setting. The lengthy duration of survival of the dementing person in the community confronts both the family and home care services with some hard decisions.

3.   DEPRESSION

This cross-national comparison of the frequency and associations of depression has included a wide range of concepts of depression: expressions of sadness, pessimism, suicidal feelings; scales whose content includes the typical symptoms of clinical depression but where the lower scores reflect a variety of common life-dissatisfactions; a latent class or statistical category of depression which is composed of roughly equal parts of demoralization syndromes (situational depression) and clinical syndromes of depression; pervasive depression, a criterion-based diagnosis which identifies cases of sufficient severity to warrant the attention of a clinician; and manic-depressive disorder (major affective disorder), the most severe and endogenous (biological) member of the depressive spectrum. The most useful indicators of depression for the cross-national comparison were the scale of depression and the pervasive category; the scale because the distribution of scores at all levels of severity could be examined across the whole of the samples and the pervasive category because it has clearcut relevance to health and social service utilization.

There was no significant difference in the frequency of depression between the elderly populations of the two cities on either the rational scale or the pervasive category of depression. This finding was contrary to our expectation that a subjective state such as depression would be extremely sensitive to cross-national variation in culture, use of language, life-style, attitudes to aging and tendencies towards stoicism or plaintiveness. We particularly noted features of life in New York which seemed more stressful and depressing for the elderly than life in London: higher crime rate, greater cost of medical care, more financial disadvantage, more environmental deprivation (inadequacies in housing), a lower proportion of elderly living in their own houses, greater heterogeneity of groups in the neighborhood, a higher rate of hospitalization, and greater problems with language barriers. Beyond these undesirable features which were confirmed by the data of this study, were stereotypes of the relative tranquility and security of old age in London. However, a closer examination of the data shows that New York does not have a monopoly of distressing events. Physical illness, disability and dependence, probably the major determinants of depression in the elderly, were of similar frequency in the two cities as was isolation and transiency of domicile.

Also evening out the impact of the environments in the two cities is the frequent discrepancy between the actual and perceived situation. Fear of crime and complaints of a deteriorating or changing neighborhood were of comparable frequency in the two cities although the respective situations actually occurred more often in New York. Correspondingly, although New Yorkers complained about deficiencies in housing more than did the Londoners, more objective itemized information showed that Londoners had more than a fair share of inadequate heating, outside toilets and poor kitchen equipment.

Similarities between the cities with respect to depression went beyond overall rates to include variation in rates or mean scores with rising age and other demographic factors: among the white groups the rates tended to go up with age in elderly males and down in females; rates were higher in females than in males; lower in those still married and in the more advantaged (in finances and environment) groups; and raised in those groups reporting fear of crime in neighborhood (43). Contrary to popular belief, living alone and current isolation (fewer social contacts) were not associated with depression in either city. Nor was there a relationship of importance with dementia scores (none in London, very low in New York). Over a broad range of situations and events, the elderly in the two cities seem to share a similar emotional response.

The age and sex patterns of depression observed in this study are consistent with those found in studies of suicide rates in age cross-sections of the population in most countries; although there is a confound between the effects of increasing age and those of successive generations (or cohorts). Another study by U.S.-U.K. Project members based on secondary analysis of national data indicates a falling rate of suicide in successively later generations of elderly white males giving a false impression in cross-section data of rates rising with age (63).

The pervasively depressed group of subjects show an increased use of medical services in both cities: they take more psychotropic medications and are given multiple drugs more often (104); they see their doctors repeatedly, receive more special investigations and are admitted to hospitals more frequently. Nevertheless, little in the way of specific treatment for depression is seen in London and even less in New York. There is clearly more than sufficient contact with the medical services but opportunities for more vigorous treatment of depression are probably being missed, especially in New York.

The comparable rates and associations of depression in the two cities and the paucity of treatment given it might lead one to expect a corresponding and cross-nationally equivalent degree of chronicity in this condition. One year follow-up results were based on numbers of cases classified as latent class depression at initial and follow-up interview. By this token and contrary to expectations, chronic cases (positive at both points in time) were twice as common in New York (15.1%) as in London (7.6%). Mean scores on the homogeneous scale of depression improved in London (4.1 to 3.2) but did not in New York (4.6 to 4.9). On the other hand, the mortality rate of the cases of pervasive depression was higher in London (10.2%) than in New York (6.9%) and this trend in mortality rates remained even when

cases of depression who were not disabled or dependent were
analysed. Given the uncertain effects of attrition due to
non-response and mortality, the results do not show a clear
advantage to either city in the outcome of pervasive
depression.

4.   DISABILITY

     The psychiatric relevance of disability in old age
stems from the role that psychiatric disorder, especially
dementia, may play in causing disability (5), and also from
the potentially stressful effect of the disability on the
individual and on others, particularly the supporting family
(6). Where the disability overwhelms the coping capacity of
the individual, of family or friends and of the
community-based health services, the risk looms large of
permanent admission to a long term care facility.

     The measure of disability used here is based on the
extent to which there is impairment of the person's ability
to care for himself in an independent fashion (5). The key
functions in this respect include the basic activities of
daily living (dressing, walking, feeding, etc.), the
instrumental activities that maintain a self-sufficient
household (shopping, cooking, cleaning, etc.) and the proper
use of community facilities (getting to the bank or the
doctor, etc.). When these adaptive abilities are lost, the
individual will no longer be able to maintain a decent
life-style at home; unless someone else more able is willing
to help by making their time available to take over some or
all of the essential tasks of survival, for free or for a fee.
The more incapacitated an individual, the more time will be
required from another in support. We assessed the duration,
frequency and level of skill of services given in support of
each incapacitated subject and thus developed a measure of
'personal time dependency' (5). Within this category we
recognized three levels of severity analogous to support
services received in a nursing home, an old age home, or from
a home care agency. The rational scale of immobility, the
homogeneous scale of activities limitation, and the category
of personal time dependency were highly related in concept
and content and statistically.

     The prevalence rates of disability were surprisingly
similar in the two cities. Mean scale scores were not
significantly different cross-nationally and about 30% of the
community elderly 65 years and older were personal time
dependent in each city. Considering that disability is the
final common pathway of a multitude of conditions (such as
dementia, stroke, heart disease, arthritis, unsteadiness,
poor vision, respiratory disease or foot problems) it is
remarkable that the results turn out so similar in the two

cities. One might have thought that probable cross-national differences in genetic predisposition, climate, diet, smoking, and other health habits would produce corresponding differences in the frequency of disability. For example, we noted that there was a greater frequency of smoking, respiratory disease and deafness in London than in New York.

We also would have expected that cross-national differences in the standards and availability of health and social care for the elderly would have led to corresponding differences in rates of disability. The elderly in London have more ready access to primary care physicians and to home care agency services than in New York; moreover, skilled nursing home beds are proportionately more numerous in New York than in London suggesting a relative bias towards institutional care in the former city. These facts can, however, be misleading: this study showed that although more Londoners had an assigned primary care physician, it was the New Yorkers who more often consulted their doctor and were intensively treated; while the later U.S.-U.K. Institutional Study (25) showed that numbers of long term care beds occupied by disabled elderly were proportionately fairly equal in the two cities, though these beds were labelled mostly as nursing home type in New York but variously found in geriatric hospitals, psychiatric hospitals and local authority (old age) homes in London.

Nevertheless, we did confirm that considerably more of the disabled and dependent elderly received formal home care services in London than in New York. The reason that the greater home care services in London did not allow that community to carry more severe and a larger proportion of disabled elderly than was the case in New York appears to be that the family (usually daughters or spouses) were more active in supporting the New York than the London elderly. Taken together, the informal (mostly families) and formal (mostly home care agencies) systems supported the same proportion of disabled elderly in the communities of the two cities. If anything, the dependent elderly in the New York community were more often severely disabled than those in London; this view is reinforced by the higher rates of mortality over the ensuing year in New York (16.2%) than in London (6.1%) among the dependent elderly, after excluding the pervasive dementias (20).

It is likely that formal services are not solicited where strong resources in the family suffice for the support of the elderly person, but it is tempting to see in these data an interplay between formal home care services and family support whereby the latter is, in some cases, displaced by the former. It is striking that although the overall rate of disability was similar, the rate among the elderly who lived alone was higher in London than in New York. It may be that formal home care has most impact in retaining the elderly in the communities where there is no family as an alternative means of support.

The vigor of the family response to the disabled elderly New Yorker was evident particularly among the black, Hispanic and Italian groups and among the more socio-economically disadvantaged classes, insofar as these groups contained the highest relative proportions of disabled elderly. It is impossible to say from these data whether these groups have an unusual capacity for coping with dependency or whether they are unable to gain access to alternative arrangements. However, a concentration of the burden of dependency among specific ethnic or religious groups and the less advantaged classes is not evident in London suggesting a more equitable distribution of support effort than appears in New York.

In both cities, the elderly who were personal time dependent were more depressed than those who were independent; perhaps the most pertinent evidence that their quality of life had deteriorated. Yet, the association of depression with dependency was less marked in the London than in the New York elderly. Possibly this is explained by the lesser severity of dependency in London than in New York but it might also suggest that the Londoners derive a greater sense of comfort from the health and social services than is the case in New York. Further clues in this direction come from the findings that Londoners, compared with New Yorkers, worry less about their health and the costs of health care, know they have a doctor they can turn to if necessary (even though they see doctors less), are less likely to be admitted to a hospital if ill, are more likely to have a protective attitude to their doctors (such as putting off seeing the doctor so as not to bother him), and are less dissatisfied with their medical treatment. It may be that a sense of confidence in the potential response of the health and social services is just as important as the actual efforts of those services.

Despite the greater activity of formal community support services in London, the dependent elderly actually receive less in the way of total (formal and informal combined) support services in London than in New York as measured by the frequency and duration of such services; analogous to the less intensive medical treatment and investigations in London than in New York.

There is a fine line to be drawn between, on the one hand, giving the elderly person a sense of support and, on the other hand, fostering dependency. There were no cross-national differences in the elderly subjects' range of motion, mobility or activity limitation. Yet the London subjects regarded themselves as being less able to look after their feet without help from a podiatrist, and less able to manage household chores than did New Yorkers; it is probable that the more ready availability of these services in London is accompanied by a greater willingness to acknowledge a need for them. The realistic acceptance by the elderly person of their own limitations and of the services offered could be seen as a beneficial health practice. However, it was notable that in London there were proportionately fewer markedly dependent elderly than found in New York. This raises the possibility that the elderly in London may more readily enter the formal home care service than in New York but also be more readily transferred out of the home care service and into institutions when they become more severely dependent. Moreover, the U.S.-U.K. Institutional Study showed that the severity of disability among the elderly in long term care facilities was probably comparable between the two cities but, if anything, greater in New York than in London (25).

Mortality rates among the dependent elderly were, as already mentioned, higher in New York than in London. However, among the survivors, chronicity and change scores as measured on the homogeneous scales of ambulation problems and activity limitation were similar in the two cities.

It appears from these data that both cities face comparable challenges in maintaining the frail elderly in the community. The response to this challenge has been somewhat different in the two cities with respect to the delivery of medical, social and home care services and with respect to the role of the family. However, the numbers and severity of cases with disability residing in the communities of the two cities remain much the same. It is likely that planners and providers of long term care services must cope with an elderly population in which roughly 30% are personal time dependent to some extent; with about equal thirds of those dependent requiring support equivalent to that found in nursing home and in old age homes and with the remaining third requiring occasional and less intensive assistance. Simple arithmetic suggests that the <u>severely</u> disabled elderly in the community outnumber those in long term care facilities by at least two-fold. The great majority of these severely disabled cases are being looked after by daughters and spouses without the assistance of formal home care services in either city. It is clear that the responsibility for the support of the severely disabled elderly is borne primarily by family members and not formal services. The toll that this takes of the family is evidenced by New York data that show the high rates of clinical depression among the elderly family members who live in the same household as a dependent elderly person (5).

Efforts to increase the proportion of disabled elderly who remain in the community as opposed to institutions must take into account that (1) families are already looking after the majority of severely disabled elderly, (2) the substantially greater activity of London home care services, and other alternatives to institutional care such as day hospitals as we note from a later U.S.-U.K. study (37, 38), is not accompanied by a greater proportion of disabled elderly in the community, (3) the supporting family is under stress, (4) formal services may in certain cases displace the family's role in caring for the elderly person, and (5) the severely disabled are only one-third of the elderly who require some level of personal assistance.

It is possible that home care services could be most effective by making the family rather than the disabled person their primary mode of intervention and including in the repertoire of home care skills the capacity to provide a feeling of support for the family and dependent elderly in addition to more material services. However, there are disabled elderly who do not have family or friends who can assist them; home care services may well be most effective and cause least erosion of independence in these cases. The success of home care services in keeping the elderly out of institutions and preserving the quality of their lives in the community may thus depend on these services extending their understanding of the psychosocial issues involved in dependency of the elderly.

5.   IMAGES AND REALITIES

At the outset of this study we shared prevailing notions that in London, as compared with New York, it is more graceful to grow old, the community tenure of the elderly is better preserved in the face of disability, and the treatment of geriatric health and social problems is more intense and effective. In short, that an older person in London is justified in feeling more supported than in New York by the community and the health and social services. These images are to some extent inconsistent with the realities of the data collected in this and related U.S.-U.K. Project studies.

As it turned out, New York does not have a monopoly of potentially stressful aspects of life for the elderly and in any case, health status and functional independence are the strongest determinants of demoralization or depression rather than the environment. Even with respect to these physical factors, the elderly in both cities show a remarkable capacity to adapt as evidenced by their equal and relatively low rates of depression.

Nor are the health and social services in London able to keep proportionately more disabled elderly outside of institutions than is the case in New York. Both cities maintain many more demented and many more disabled elderly out of institutions than inside of them. A little less than a third of the elderly population in both cities are receiving some level of personal assistance to maintain themselves in the community; about 10% or less of the elderly population are as disabled as those in nursing homes. It is true that the delivery of home care services in London is much more active than in New York but families in New York make up the difference.

Although there are more health services formally identified as geriatric in London than in New York, it is the elderly in the latter city who more often see their doctors, are given special investigations and receive highly potent medications. The elderly with pervasive depression receive much psychotropic medication in both cities but few are given specific antidepressants and seldom are psychiatrists directly involved in their treatment: nevertheless, depressives in London do receive more specific treatment than in New York. In neither city do cases of dementia receive much in the way of psychotropic medication, probably an advantage over the practice in institutions. All in all, there is no dramatic picture favoring the delivery of more intensive geriatric treatment in London.

Yet, the elderly in London do seem to have a more supportive image of their health and social services than is the case in New York. Almost all the London elderly claim to have a doctor and to expect to receive a housecall if they needed it; they are more likely to be treated at home instead of in hospitals when ill; they are less dissatisfied with the treatment they received and less likely to avoid treatment because of lack of confidence in the care system or because of cost. The London elderly are in general less worried and concerned about their health and less inclined to develop depression in association with physical illnes and dependence. They even seem protective of the health services insofar as they sometimes put off seeing the doctor if they think he has more urgent cases to attend to; a sentiment almost never expressed by New Yorkers.

The overarching impression gained from the cross-national comparisons discussed here is that the health and social problems of the elderly in the two cities are more similar than dissimilar but the health and social services have cross-nationally differing styles and emphases. There is no clear evidence in this study that the management of depression, dementia or disability in the community is dramatically better in one or the other city though there is some edge in favor of the formal primary care and home care services in London and specialist care and the family role in New York. In view of the complexity of the problems and of their management, it is not surprising that no dramatic cross-nationally differential impact of services on community tenure and prevalence of health problems is discernible. There is carried in these findings a clear caution against expecting that simply a greater volume of service activity, such as increased home care services, will necessarily visibly alter the rates of institutional admission.

These are not arguments to do less about these disorders of old age but rather that an effective health and social service response requires great understanding of the interplay of disorders of health with service systems and community supports. Given the uncertainties of the effects of new service initiatives it would seem best for the present to plan systems of care which have flexibility and a variety of options for care and not to bank too heavily on a particular emphasis.

The search for approaches to care of the elderly which have more predictable effects than exists currently, should not be restricted to the more tangible effects such as preventing unnecessary distress, chronicity, decline and institutional admission. The psychological effects of services, particularly the projection of an image which makes the elderly person feel reassured and supported with respect to health and associated social problems, is of great importance. In this area the London system of care seemed to have the advantage over New York. The supportive image may be of value not only in encouraging an adaptation to health problems, but also in improving the quality of life of the elderly who are in good health but must consider their prospects should they fall ill. It may also be that services that are seen as supportive will be more wisely used by potential clients.

It is tempting to close by further contrasting the features of London and New York services that might relate to the projection of a supportive image. However, it is the function of a study such as this to suggest potentially fruitful lines of analysis, speculation and additional investigation but not to expect closure on the issues. It is therefore appropriate that the report of the U.S.-U.K. Geriatric Community Study should end where the answers and the questions that the data provide have been clarified.

Appendix I

Subject Identification:

Date:

			✓ IF QUOTA FILLED	
			Quota = 1	Quota = 2
A.	LIMITED DEPRESSION	✓ IF PRESENT		
	1 Depression lasts only a few hours - can snap out of it	1( )		
	2 Occasional low days	2( )		
	3 Worried about specific problem - can turn mind to other things	3( )		
	4 Cries only when a particular event or situation is discussed	4( )		
	5 Future looks empty	5( )		

B.	PERVASIVE DEPRESSION			
	1 Depression lasts whole day or longer	1( )		
	2 Cries or feels like crying, often	2( )		
	3 Depression is bothersome and not easily shaken off	3( )		
	4 Future looks bleak or unbearable	4( )		
	5 Can't stop worrying - worry is disproportionate to cause	5( )		
	6 Looks depressed through much of interview	6( )		

C.	VEGETATIVE SYMPTOMS (Not accounted for by physical disease)			
	1 Palpitations	1( )		
	2 Trembling	2( )		
	3 Dizziness	3( )		
	4 Poor appetite	4( )		
	5 Constipation	5( )		
	6 Loss of weight	6( )		
	7 Sleep disturbance	7( )		
	8 Poor concentration	8( )		
	9 Early morning awakening	9( )		
	10 Lies awake with anxious or depressing thoughts	10( )		
	11 Depression worst in mornings	11( )		
	12 Weak or tired	12( )		
	13 Slow in speech or movement	13( )		
	14 Unexplained aches and pains	14( )		
	15 Subjective complaints of impaired memory	15( )		

CRITERIA FOR DIAGNOSIS AND
SEVERITY OF DEPRESSION (continued)

Subject Identification:

Date:

D. SELF-DEPRECIATION	√ IF PRESENT	√ IF QUOTA FILLED Quota = 1
1 Self-conscious in public	1( )	
2 Feels a failure	2( )	
3 Feels guilty	3( )	

E. SUICIDAL OR PSYCHOTIC (Not accounted for
by a non-depressive state)

1 Actively suicidal (strong impulse, preparations, or attempt)	1( )	
2 Deluded or hallucinated with a depressive content	2( )	
3 Mute or immobile	3( )	
4 Serious injury or ill effect following suicidal attempt	4( )	
5 Starvation or intercurrent infection	5( )	
6 Homicidal behavior	6( )	

F. OTHER FEATURES

1 Stress: a. Irrelevant ( )	
b. Necessary ( ) or Sufficient ( )	
c. Concurrent ( ) or Precedent ( )	
2 Current or Past Excitement:	Yes ( ) No ( )
3 Present Episode:	Yes ( ) No ( )
4 Past Episode:	Yes ( ) No ( )
5 Positive Mood:	Yes ( ) No ( )

RULES FOR RATING CRITERIA FOR DIAGNOSIS
AND SEVERITY OF DEPRESSION

General

In making the ratings take into account all information in the
summary (with only the explicit diagnosis expurgated), and the
profile of rational scores. Where inadequate information is
provided in a summary the following note should be applied: A
high score on depression (11+) and a quota score on Section B
allows one to add one point assigned to any item in Section C
(thus the C quota may be fulfilled in this way).

> Not to be considered in making ratings (even where known)
> are the following:

>> Treatment received
>> Self-labeling
>> Symptoms which are 'suspected' rather than
>>   reported or observed
>> The diagnosis of the rater who wrote the summary

> Time: Rate only symptoms that occurred in past month (unless
>   otherwise specified).

>   Example - If two months ago the subject had a
>   Pervasive Depression but over the past month it was a
>   Limited Depression (at worst) then it qualifies as a
>   Limited Depression.

If symptoms fluctuated over past month then rate them at their
worst, except that the depression must occur in more than one
week of the month to qualify as Limited and in more than two
weeks to qualify as Pervasive.

> Positive mood is rated at best in past month.

> Transient situational neuroses can qualify as Limited
> Depression if they last one week or more.

> Don't count habitual constipation preceding the depression.

A.   Limited Depression

> As defined in the criteria. In general it refers to
> depression which is transient or can be self suppressed so
> that a substantial part of life is free of depression. The
> severity of depression while it lasts is not an issue; nor
> is the response of the person to antidepressant medication;
> nor past history.

By definition, vegetative signs and attempted suicide (for example) may occur in Limited Depression. Where there is difficulty in deciding between Limited and Pervasive Depression, the presence of positive mood sways the diagnosis toward the former diagnosis; so does a low depression score (<6) or the presence of good life satisfaction or a self rating of being very happy. The low score and self-ratings may also decide the diagnosis against even Limited Depression in cases of doubt. Conversely, it may be borne in mind that cases with a score of 6 or more on depression (rational scales) may have either Limited or Pervasive Depression.

B.   Pervasive Depression

As defined in the criteria. In general it refers to depression that pervades most aspects of life.

Depression that occurs regularly each day for a large portion of the day and at the same time of day (e.g., morning) is regarded as qualifying for B3 - "Depression is bothersome and not easily shaken off."

If several (four or more) symptoms are rated in Sections B through E, with only one occurring in B then Pervasive Depression should be rated nonetheless.

C.   Vegetative Symptoms

A judgment must be made whether the symptoms germane to this area are due to psychiatric or medical causes. The latter do not qualify whereas the former do. A note on memory appears below. With respect to the other vegetative symptoms bear in mind that vegetative symptoms are likely to be psychiatric if:

1.   there is no accompanying physical illness

2.   the symptoms are undiagnosed or are diagnosed as "due to nerves," etc.

3.   the symptoms are preceded by a feeling of anxiety

4.   wakefulness (i.e., sleep disturbance) is accompanied by depressing or anxious thoughts rather than pain, etc.

5.   early morning wakening occurs (wakes two or more hours before usual time and wants to go back to sleep but cannot)

On the other hand, tiredness occurring as a result if long hours at work or unusual effort is not rated as psychiatric; nor is weight loss due to dieting, symptoms caused by medications, shortened sleep hours without difficulty in falling asleep or tiredness on wakening.

Sleep Disturbance

Sleep disturbance with the distinctive pattern of depression (See 4 and 5 above) rates in two places (Sections C7 and C9 or C10). Early morning wakening should not be rated unless the subject wants to go back to sleep (feels the need for more sleep) and yet cannot. Under these circumstances early morning wakening also counts as sleep disturbance (i.e., picks up two points).

Memory

Subjective complaints of impaired memory refers to the subjects report; never to the rater's observations or tests. The performance testing of memory shows little or no impairment. Typically the subject complains of difficulty in remembering names (but not of close friends or family), misplacing possessions, being muddled about appointments, forgetting what they were intending to do, forgetting something just seen or heard, and difficulty in recalling the right word to use in phrasing a thought, or getting thoughts mixed up.

D. Self-depreciation

As defined in criteria.

E. Suicidal or Psychotic

As defined in criteria.

F. Other Features

Stress

Stress is irrelevant if it does not appear to explain the depression (see below); necessary if it has played a substantial part in causing the depression but is not overwhelming (i.e., many people are not depressed in those circumstances); sufficient if it is overwhelming and would cause depression in most people. An example of sufficient stress would be a recent bereavement; or a previously active and energetic person being rendered severely handicapped in a relatively short period of time.

If stress is necessary or sufficient then it must be classified as precedent when the depression follows the stress and concurrent if the depression is accompanied by ongoing stress. Bereavement is regarded as a precedent

stress.   Depression   associated   with   disability   or
environmental deprivation is concurrent.   A judgment must
be made in other cases as to whether it is an event or its
consequences that is the stress (the former is precedent
and the latter is concurrent).   Where this is difficult to
judge   the   following   arbitrary   rule   should   be   used:
Depression which outlasts an event by one year becomes
concurrent - by five years is free-floating.

Irrelevant Stress

Irrelevant stress is to be rated when there is no apparent
stress to account for the depression; or when the stress
that is suggested by the subject is implausible (e.g.,
trivial); or when there have been a series of depressions
each with a different cause attributed to it (i.e., almost
anything triggers the depression), or when a variety of
events   such   as   past   bereavements,   relocations   and
retirement have changed the subject's life style to one
which though not acutely deprived is viewed negatively by
the subject.

Positive Mood

Refers to the following features:

Cheerful most of interview; pleasant and well groomed;
seeks social activities and contacts; mentions enjoyable
activities; mentions positive attitudes.

CLASSIFICATION OF DEPRESSION

1. SEVERITY CRITERIA:

```
A                 Level 1
B                 Level 2
B + (C or D) = Level 3
B + (C +  D) = Level 4
B + E        = Level 5
```

2. CLASSIFICATION:

```
A                       = Limited Depression
B in any combination = Pervasive Depression
C in the absence of B = Masked Depression
```

3. SUBCLASSIFICATION OF PERVASIVE DEPRESSION:

```
B + Irrelevant Stress = Free-floating Depression
B + Sufficient Stress = Reactive Depression
B + Necessary Stress  = Aggravated Depression
```

```
B + Precedent Stress = Subsequent Depression
B + Concurrent Stress = Concurrent Depression
```

4. TRANSLATION INTO CONVENTIONAL DIAGNOSTIC LABELS

Manic-depressive - depressive disorder is operationally
defined as (B) pervasive depression + (C) vegetative
symptoms + insufficient stress (i.e., other than
sufficient) + episodes (present or past).

Appendix II

<u>CRITERIA FOR DIAGNOSIS AND SEVERITY OF DEMENTIA</u>

Subject Identification:

Date:

✓ IF QUOTA FILLED

A. LIMITED COGNITIVE DISTURBANCE	✓ IF PRESENT	Quota = 1	Quota = 2
1 Reports a decline in memory	1( )		
2 Increased reliance on notes as reminders	2( )		
3 Occasionally (less than once a week) forgets names of acquaintances, or forgets appointments or misplaces objects	3( )		
4 Occasionally (less than once a month) has destructive or dangerous memory lapses such as burning cooking or leaving on gas tap	4( )		
5 One or two errors on cognitive testing: forgets current or past president, exact date, phone number, zip code, dates of moving to present location; can't remember interviewer's name even on third challenge	5( )		

B. PERVASIVE COGNITIVE DISTURBANCE

1 Frequently shows lapses in A3	1( )		
2 More than two errors in A5	2( )		
3 Keeps forgetting important or recent events even after repeated reminders	3( )		
4 Forgets name of close friends or family or other frequent contacts and cannot soon correct self	4( )		
5 Has at least once in past month forgotten the way home from a point in neighborhood	5( )		
6 Several years out in age, birth or present year	6( )		

C. DEPENDENT

1 Frequently (at least once a week) forgets familiar contexts, i.e., acts as if he is in a different context (as at work), at a different age (still a young person), or with a different person (Misidentifies interviewer as close family member and doesn't correct self)	1( )		

CRITERIA FOR DIAGNOSIS AND
SEVERITY OF DEMENTIA (continued)

Subject Identification:

Date:

		√ IF QUOTA FILLED	
C. DEPENDENT (continued) √ IF PRESENT		Quota = 1	Quota = 2
2 Wanders; gets lost frequently (at least once a month) or is restricted or escorted because of wandering	2( )		
3 Shows indiscreet behavior (e.g., undresses in public, lights fires, steals	3( )		
4 Panics if alone	4( )		
5 Puttering about most of the night	5( )		
6 Apathetic and largely inactive during day	6( )		
7 Requires supervision for administration of medication	7( )		
8 Requires supervision for bathing and eating	8( )		

D. REGRESSED (not accounted for by a physical disorder)

1 Incontinent (less than once a month) of feces or urine	1( )	
2 Has to be taken to toilet regularly to avoid accidents	2( )	
3 Only communication is of basic needs or empty social forms	3( )	
4 Irrelevant or stock answers to fairly simple questions	4( )	
5 Requires to be dressed, washed or groomed	5( )	
6 Requires to be fed	6( )	

E. DETERIORATED (Not accounted for by a physical disorder)

1 Bed or chairbound or cannot move wheelchair	1( )	
2 Has to be transferred	2( )	
3 Doubly and frequently incontinent or on catheter	3( )	
4 Utterances are unintelligible	4( )	
5 Doesn't communicate needs	5( )	
6 Unresponsive	6( )	

CRITERIA FOR DIAGNOSIS AND
SEVERITY OF DEMENTIA (continued)

Subject Identification:

Date:

F.	OTHER FEATURES		Yes	No
1	Positive Cognition		( )	( )
2	Supervision required		( )	( )
3	Progressive over last five years		( )	( )
4	Duration: Over five years		( )	( )
5	Six months to five years	or	( )	( )
6	Less than six months		( )	( )
7	MSQ: Moderately impaired		( )	( )
8	Grossly impaired	or	( )	( )
9	Lucid intervals during past six months		( )	( )
10	Last less than one week	or	( )	( )
11	Last one week or more		( )	( )
12	Evidence of Arteriosclerosis		( )	( )
13	Episodes occur in last five years		( )	( )
14	Episodes coincide: With general illness or medication		( )	( )
15	With relocation or other stress		( )	( )
16	Misperceptions or hallucinations		( )	( )
17	Marked tremor or stiffness or other Parkinsonian feature		( )	( )
18	Above preceded onset of cognitive disturbance by 3 years or more		( )	( )

RULES FOR RATING CRITERIA FOR DIAGNOSIS
AND SEVERITY OF DEMENTIA

General

In making the ratings take into account all information in the
case summary (with only the explicit psychiatric diagnosis
expurgated), and the profile of rational scores.

> Time: Rate only symptoms in past month (unless otherwise
> specified). If symptoms fluctuated during the past
> month then rate at worst, except positive cognition is
> rated at best in past month.

A.   Limited Cognitive Disturbance

As defined in the criteria. Refers usually to an
impairment of memory but with substantial aspects of living
adequately performed, e.g., memory lapses but positive
cognition as well or memory lapses but largely independent
(requiring little or no supervision).

B.-E. Pervasive Cognitive Disturbance

As defined in the criteria. Refers usually to an
impairment of memory which renders the subject incapable of
certain task performance (ADL-IADL) and renders it
necessary for the subject to be supervised (see
Supervision). Levels B, C, D and E as defined in the
criteria.

F.   Other Features:

Positive Cognition - Refers to a capacity which would be
surprising to find in one who is demented such as the
following:

- Able to go out alone and beyond immediate neighborhood
  (e.g., to church, cinema), and finds way back safely.
  Can use public transportation alone. Able to stay in
  unfamiliar accommodation without resulting confusion.

- Shops or cooks without aid (or performs other
  complicated task).

- Lives alone.

- Able to conduct a rich and varied and responsive
  conversation which is full of accurate facts - can
  relate an internally consistent and complicated
  chronology of recent events such as operations,

relocations (sequence correct even if dates are imprecise) - can discuss current events and abstract a conclusion from them - can relate the story of a recent book read or film seen.

- Takes an active interest in a social network and keeps track of those in it. (Not merely being cheerful and putting on a good social manner, which is positive for mood).

- Can describe a complicated personal situation (e.g., dealings with a public agency, the course and treatment of an illness, details of medication, etc.).

- Looking after a sick spouse.

- Involved in hobbies which require ability and the capacity to follow written instructions.

- Anticipatory knowledge of an imminent future event not of a routine nature (e.g., a visit or excursion).

- Able to carry on a written correspondence without help.

Supervision

Refers to the need for someone to supervise, assist or substitute for subject in performing tasks under cognitive control. These are continence, housekeeping, cooking, dressing, handling money and business, shopping, initiative and planning, and needing to be accompanied on excursions to avoid wandering, etc. If there is a physical disability requiring personal intervention the latter does not count as supervision. If it is not clear whether the need for supervision is physical or cognitive then 'supervision' is rated positive. Do not include assistance or supervision in response to the subject's anxiety about excursions (agoraphobia).

Certain deficits in the subject are specifically suggestive of poor cognitive control: incontinence without awareness; wandering; loss of ability to manage cash; forgetting what to buy when in shop, etc. Certain other deficits are suggestive of non-cognitive causes: inability to do heavy chores, carry heavy parcels, etc.

Supervision is most clearly seen when someone has made special arrangements to provide it (e.g., a formal service, given up job to do so, moved in with subject, given up going out so as not to leave subject alone, etc.).

Progressive - There has been a definite deterioration visible at least over a five year or lesser period.

Moderate vs. Gross MSQ Errors - Gross errors are (1) total disorientation for time (not even approximately right in day, month, year, age), (2) high MSQ scores (8 + on rational scale).

Moderate includes (1) giving an incorrect answer on MSQ but correcting it either spontaneously or on challenge, or (2) a low score on MSQ (2-4), or (3) an intermediate score on MSQ (5-7) but in a person with poor education or (4) an error-free MSQ score (0-1) but errors in giving other facts and dates (e.g., date of marriage).

Lucid Intervals - An apparent return to normal cognition.

Evidence of Arteriosclerosis - Should be rated when the subject with pervasive memory disturbance: (1) Has hypertension and a series of 'blackouts' (but not if the blackouts only occur on rising from sitting or lying to a standing position, and not if hypertension alone nor blackouts alone, and not dizziness). (2) Has a series of unexplained falls not explained by weakness or tripping (and not dizziness alone). (3) Episodes of time in which speech is lost or disrupted, dysarthria, slurred speech, there is weakness or paralysis on one side (stroke), incoordination; especially if an episode or series of episodes precede the memory disturbance.

Do not include a diagnosis by a doctor of hardening of the arteries or arteriosclerosis.

Do not include leg cramps on walking (intermittent claudication), tremors, dysphasia (e.g., difficulty with naming objects). Where in doubt between arteriosclerosis and senile dementia diagnose the latter.

Episodes - the symptoms described for dementia have had at least one distinct onset and termination during the past five years.

Coincide with General Illness or Medication - Refers to episodes of cognitive disturbances which appear to have an onset and termination related to an acute illness (e.g., infection, dehydration, acute cardiac failure) or a potent medication (e.g., barbiturate, antidepressant).

Misperceptions or Hallucinations - Has visual hallucinations (e.g., sees objects that aren't there) or misperceptions (e..g, sees stable objects moving). These misperceptions or hallucinations are not considered if they occur only when the person is falling asleep.

Onset Preceded by Insult to Brain - Immediately before the onset of the cognitive disturbance there was some injury to the brain due to accident, lack of oxygen (e.g., cardiac arrest), infection (e.g., encephalitis), or spread of cancer, etc. Stroke is excluded as this is rated under arteriosclerosis.

Parkinsonian Features - Marked tremor of hands and a stiff shuffling gait sufficient to disable the subject to some extent or treatment with L-Dopa or other anti-Parkinsonian drug (e.g., Cogentin). Exclude side effects of major tranquilizers.

CLASSIFICATION OF DEMENTIA

1.   SEVERITY CRITERIA:

        A   Level 1
        B   Level 2
        B* + C   = Level 3
        (B* or C) + D = Level 4
        (B* or C) + E = Level 5

        *If the subject is too sick to test B, then Level 3-5 must
        be based either on a history of B or on C, D, or E alone.

2.   CLASSIFICATION:

        Limited Cognitive Disturbance = Level 1; or Level 2 +
        Positive Cognition.

        Pervasive Dementia = Level 2 without Positive Cognition, or
        Level 3-5.

3.   SUBCLASSIFICATION OF PERVASIVE DEMENTIA:

        i. Arteriosclerotic Dementia - evidence of arterioscle-
           rosis as defined elsewhere.

       ii. Acute Confusional State - no evidence of arterioscle-
           rosis.   Episodes coincide with general illness or
           medication.
           - Lucid intervals.
           - Duration less than six months.
           - Misperceptions or hallucinations.

      iii. Secondary Dementia - no evidence of above (i) and
           (ii).
           - Onset preceded immediately by insult to brain, or
           - Evidence of Parkinson's Disease preceding cogni-
             tive disturbance by three or more years.

       iv. Senile (Alzheimer's) Dementia - no evidence of above
           states (i-iii).
           - Duration less than 10 years.
           - Visible progress over past 5 years.
           - No lucid interval lasting over 1 week, in past
             6 months.
           - Marked fluctuations do not occur unless the
             episodes of deterioration occur with illness,
             medication, relocation or stress.

        v. Unclassified: the residual cases of Pervasive Cogni-
           tive Disturbance.

Bibliography

Papers on the U.S.-U.K. Cross-National
Geriatric Community Study

1. Gurland, B.J. Aims, organization, and initial studies of the Cross-National Project. International Journal of Aging & Human Development, 7, pp. 283-293, 1976.
2. Dean, L., Teresi, J., and Wilder, D. The human element in survey research. In: International Journal of Aging & Human Development, 8, pp. 83-92, 1977.
3. Gurland, B.J., Copeland, J.R.M., Sharpe, L., Kelleher, M.J., Kuriansky, J.B., and Simon, R. Assessment of the older person in the community. International Journal of Aging & Human Development, 8, pp. 1-8, 1977.
4. Gurland, B.J., Kuriansky, J.B., Sharpe, L., Simon, R., Stiller, P., and Birkett, P. The Comprehensive Assessment and Referral Evaluation (CARE) - Rationale, development and reliability. International Journal of Aging & Human Development, 8, pp. 9-42, 1977.
5. Gurland, B., Dean, L., Gurland, R., and Cook, D. Personal time dependency in the elderly of New York City. In: Dependency in the Elderly of N.Y.C. Community Council of Greater New York, October, 1978.
6. Teresi, J., Bennett, R., and Wilder, D. Personal time dependency and family attitudes. In: Dependency in the Elderly of N.Y.C. Community Council of Greater New York, October, 1978.
7. Gurland, B.J. The borderlands of dementia: The influence of socioculture characteristics on rates of dementia occurring in the senium. In: N.E. Miller and G.D. Cohen (Eds.), Clinical Aspects of Alzheimer's Disease and Senile Dementia (Aging, Vol. 15). New York: Raven Press, 1981, pp. 61-84.
8. Bennett, R. and Cook, D. Isolation of the aged in New York City. In: Planning for the Elderly in New York City. Community Council of Greater New York, April, 1980, pp. 26-42.

9. Wilder, D. The assessment of chronicity-Results of a longitudinal study. In: Proceedings of a Research Utilization Workshop. Community Council of Greater New York, April, 1980, pp.43-54.

10. Gurland, B., Dean, L., Cross, P., and Golden, R. The epidemiology of depression and dementia in the elderly: The use of multiple indicators of these conditions. In: J.E. Cole, and J.E. Barrett (Eds.), Psychopathology in the Aged. New York: Raven Press, 1980, pp. 37-60.

11. Gurland, B., Golden, R., and Dean, L. Depression and dementia in the elderly of New York City. In: Proceedings of a Research Utilization Workshop. Community Council of Greater New York, 1980.

12. Golden, R. A method for detection and testing of a conjectured latent taxon. In: Columbia University Statistical Reports. Technical Report No. 13-14, August, 1981.

13. Gurland, B. and Zubin, J. The United States-United Kingdom Cross-National Project: Issues in Cross-Cultural Psychogeriatric Research. In: L.L. Adler (Ed.), Cross-Cultural Research at Issue. New York: Academic Press, 1982 (in press).

14. Gurland, B.J., Dean, L., Copeland, J.R.M., Gurland, R., and Golden, R. Criteria for the diagnosis of dementia in the community elderly. Gerontologist, 22(2), pp. 180-186, 1982.

15. Gurland, B.J., Golden, R.R., and Challop, J. Unidimensional and multidimensional approaches to the differentiation of depression and dementia in the elderly. In: S. Corkin, S., K.L. Davis, J.H. Growden, E. Usdin and R.J. Wurtman (Eds.), Alzheimer's Disease: A Report of Progress in Research. New York: Raven Press, 1981, pp. 119-125.

16. Golden, R.R., Teresi, J.A., and Gurland, B.J. Detection of taxonomic classes of health and social problems with the indicator-scale of the C.A.R.E. Interview Schedule. Manuscript submitted for publication, 1982.

17. Golden, R.R., Teresi, J.A., and Gurland, B.J. Development and reliability of indicator-scales for the Comprehensive Assessment and Referral Evaluation Interview Schedule. Journal of Gerontology (in press).

18. Teresi, J.A., Golden, R.R., and Gurland, B.J. Construct validity of indicator-scales developed for the Comprehensive Assessment and Referral Evaluation Interview Schedule. Journal of Gerontology (in press).

19. Teresi, J.A., Golden, R.R., and Gurland, B.J. Concurrent and predictive validity of indicator-scales developed for the Comprehensive Assessment and Referral Evaluation Interview Schedule. Journal of Gerontology (in press).

20. Professional Staff of the U.S.-U.K. Cross-National Project. A report of a one-year follow-up of the elderly living in their communities in New York City and London. Unpublished manuscript, 1982 (available from authors).

21. Golden, R. A taxometric model for the detection of a conjectured latent taxon. Multivariate Behavioral Research, July 1982, Vol. 17, pp. 389-416.

22. Gurland B.J., Golden, R., Teresi, J., and Challop, J. The SHORT-CARE: An efficient instrument for the assessment of depression, dementia, and disability. Journal of Gerontology (in press).

23. Gurland, B.J., and Wilder, D.W. The "CARE" Interview Revisited: Development of an efficient, systematic clinical assessment. Journal of Gerontology (in press).

24. Golden, R., Tersei, J.A., and Gurland, B.J. Development and testing of indicator scales for the Comprehensive Assessment and Referral Evaluation Interview Schedule for the epidemiological study of health and social problems of older individuals living in the community. Unpublished manuscript, 1982 (available from authors).

Other Relevant U.S.-U.K. Cross-National Project Papers

25. Gurland, B., Cross, P., Defiguerido, J., Shannon, M., Mann, A.H., Jenkins R., Bennett, R., Wilder, D., Wright, H., Killeffer, E., and Godlove, C. A cross-national comparison of the institutionalized elderly in the cities of New York and London. Psychological Medicine, 9, pp. 781-788, 1979.

26. Godlove, C., Dunn, G., and Wright, H. Caring for old people in New York and London: The 'Nurses Aide' Interview. Journal of the Royal Society of Medicine, 73, pp. 713-723, 1980.

27. Zubin, J. and Gurland, B.J. The United States-United Kingdom project on diagnosis of the mental disorders. Annals of N.Y. Academy of Science, 285, pp. 676-686, 1977.

28. Gurland, B.J. Kuriansky, J.B., Sharpe, L., Simon, R.J., Stiller, P.R., Fleiss, J.L. (US) with Copeland, J.R.M., Kelleher, M., Gourlay, A.J., Cowan, D., and Barron, G. (UK) A comparison of the outcome of hospitalization of geriatric patients in public psychiatric wards in New York and London. Canadian Psychiatric Association Journal, 21, pp. 421-432, 1976.

29. Kuriansky, J.B., Gurland, B.J., Fleiss, M., and Cowan, D.M. The assessment of self-care capacity in geriatric psychiatric patients by objective and subjective methods. Journal of Clinical Psychology, 32, pp. 95-102, 1976.

30. Simon, R.J., Kuriansky, J.B., Fleiss, J.L., and Gurland, B.J. Pathways to the hospital for the geriatric psychiatric patient in New York and London. American Journal of Public Health, 66, pp. 1074-1077, 1976.

31. Copeland, J.R.M., Kelleher, M.J., Kellett, J.M., Fountain-Gourlay, A.J., Cowan, D.W., Barron, G., DeGruchy, J. (UK) with Gurland, B.J., Sharpe, L., Simon, R.J., Kuriansky, J., and Stiller, P. (US) Cross-national study of the diagnosis of mental disorders: A comparison of the diagnoses of elderly psychiatric patients admitted to mental hospitals serving Queens County, New York and the former borough of Camberwell, London. British Journal of Psychiatry, 126, pp. 11-20, 1975.

32. Cowan, D., Wright, P., Kelleher, M.J., Copeland, J.R.M., Kellett, J.M., Fountain-Gourlay, A.J., Barron, G., DeGruchy, J. (UK) with Kuriansky, J., Gurland, B., Sharpe, L., Simon, R., and Stiller, P. Cross-national study of diagnosis of the mental disorders: A comparative psychometric assessment of elderly patients admitted to mental hospitals serving Queens County, New York, and the Old Borough of Camberwell, London. British Journal of Psychiatry, 126, pp. 560-570, 1975.

33. Copeland, J.R.M., Kelleher, M.J., Kellett, J.M., Fountain-Gourlay, A.J., Cowan, D.W., Barron, G., Degruchy, J. (UK) with Gurland, B.J., Kuriansky, J.B., Sharpe, L., Simon, R.J., and Stiller, P.R. (US) Diagnostic differences in psychogeriatric patients in New York and London. Canadian Psychiatric Association Journal, 19, pp. 267-271, 1974.

34. Professional Staff of US & UK Cross-National Project. The diagnosis and psychopathology of schizophrenia in New York and London. Schizophrenia Bulletin, 11, Winter, pp. 80-102, 1974.

35. Fleiss, J.L., Gurland, B.J., Simon, R.J., and Sharpe, L. Cross-national study of diagnosis of the mental disorders: Some demographic correlates of hospital diagnosis in New York and London. International Journal of Social Psychiatry, 19, pp. 180-186, 1973.

36. Gurland, B., Bennett, R., and Wilder, D. Reevaluating the place of evaluation in planning for alternatives to institutional care for the elderly. In: M. Shinn and B.J. Felton (Eds.), Institutions and Alternatives. Journal of Social Issues, Vol. 37, pp. 51-68, 1981.

37. MacDonald, A.J., Mann, A.J., Jenkins, R., Richard, L., Godlove, C., and Rodwell, G. An attempt to determine the impact of four types of care upon the elderly in London by the study of matched groups. Psychological Medicine, 1982 (in press).

38. Professional Staff of US-UK Cross-National Project. A comparison of the frail elderly in day treatment of those in long term institutional care in New York City and London. Report submitted to Administration on Aging, June 1982.

39. Godlove, C., Richard, L., and Graham, R. An observation study of elderly people in four different 'care environments.' Institute of Psychiatry, London. Unpublished manuscript, 1980 (available from authors).

40. Cooper, J.E., Kendell, K.E., Gurland, B.J., Sharpe, L., Copeland, J.R.M., and Simon, R.J. Psychiatric Diagnosis in New York and London: A Comparative Study of Mental Hospital Admissions, Maudsley Monograph No. 20, Oxford University Press, London, 1972.

Papers on Depression, Dementia and Disability in the Elderly by U.S.-U.K. Cross-National Project Staff

41. Gurland, B.J. and Birkett, P. Senile and presenile Dementia. In: W. Shepard, H. Russell, and W. Lader (Eds.), Handbook of Psychiatry on Mental Disorders and Somatic Illness. Cambridge Press, 1982 (in press).

42. Gurland, B.J. Psychiatric aspects of normal aging and the pseudodementias. In: R. Mayeux and W. Rosen (Eds.), Recent Advances in Dementia. New York: Raven Press, 1982 (in press).

43. Gurland, B.J., Dean, L., and Cross, P. Effects of depression on individual social functioning in the elderly. In: Depression in the Elderly. Springer Publishing, 1982 (in press).

44. Gurland, B.J. and Toner, J.A. Depression and aging. In: C. Eisdorfer (Ed.), Annual Review of Gerontology & Geriatrics, Vol. 3, 1982, pp. 365-418.

45. Gurland, B.J. and Cross, P. The epidemiology of mental disorders in old age: Some clinical implications. In: L.F. Jarvik (Ed.), The Psychiatric Clinics of North America: Aging, Vol. 5, No. 1. April, 1982, pp. 11-26.

46. Gurland, B. The assessment of the mental health status of older adults. In: J.E. Birren and R. Sloane (Eds.), Handbook of Mental Health and Aging. Englewood Cliffs, N.J.: Prentice Hall, Inc., 1980, pp. 671-700.

47. Copeland, J.R.M. and Gurland, B.J. Evaluation of diagnostic methods: International comparison. In: F. Post (Ed.), Studies of Geriatric Psychiatry. New York: John Wiley, 1979, pp. 191-209.

48. Gurland, B.J., Bennett, R., and Wilder, D. International developments in psychogeriatric care. Generations, Vol. III, No. 4, Spring, 1979.

49. Gurland, B.J. Some considerations regarding research in the epidemiology of the mental disorders of older persons. In: Issues in Mental Health and Aging, Vol. I Research, NIMH. Proceedings of the Conference on Research in Mental Health and Aging, Nov. 10-11, 1975. Bethesda, Maryland: DHEW Publication #(ADM) 79-663, p. 39, printed in 1979.

50. Gurland, B.J. Psychiatric classification: Nosology and taxonomy. In: B. Wolman (Ed.), International Encyclopedia of Psychiatry, Psychology, Psychoanalysis & Neurology. New York: Van Nostrand Reinhold Co., 1978, Vol. 1, pp. 156-160

51. Birkett, D.P. Measuring dementia. Journal of the American Geriatric Society, 25, pp. 153-156, 1977.

52. Mulligan, M. and Bennett, R. Assessment of mental health and social problems during multiple friendly visits: The development and evaluation of a Friendly Visiting Program. International Journal of Aging & Human Development, 8, pp. 67-82, 1977.

53. Copeland, J.R.M., Kelleher, M.J., Duckworth, G., and Smith, A. Reliability of psychiatric assessment in older patients. International Journal of Aging & Human Development, 7, pp. 313-322, 1976.

54. Copeland, J.R.M., Kelleher, M.J., Kellett, J.M., Gourlay, A.J. (UK) with Gurland, B.J., Fleiss, J.L., and Sharpe, L. (US) A semi-structured clinical interview for the assessment of diagnosis and mental state in the elderly: The Geriatric Mental State Schedule. I. Development and

Reliability. Psychological Medicine, 6, pp. 439-449, 1976.

55. Fleiss, J.L., Gurland, B.J., and Des Roche, P. Distinctions between organic brain syndrome and functional psychiatric disorders: Based on the Geriatric Mental State Interivew. International Journal of Aging & Human Development, 7, pp. 323-330, 1976.

56. Gurland, B.J. The comparative frequency and types of depression in various adult age groups. Journal of Gerontology, 31, pp. 283-292, 1976.

57. Gurland, B.J., Copeland, J.R.M., Sharpe, L., and Kelleher, M.J. The Geriatric Mental Status Interview (GMS). International Journal of Aging & Human Development, 7, pp. 303-311, 1976.

58. Gurland, B.J., Fleiss, J., Goldberg, G., Sharpe, L. (US) with Copeland, J.R.M., Kelleher, M.J., and Kellett, J.M. (UK) The Geriatric Mental State Schedule II. Factor analysis. Psychological Medicine, 6, pp. 451-459, 1976.

59. Kelleher, M.J., Copeland, J.R.M., Gurland, B.J., and Sharpe, L. Assessment of the older psychiatric inpatient. International Journal of Aging & Human Development, 7, pp. 195-302, 1976.

60. Gurland, B.J. A broad clinical assessment of psychopathology in the aged. In: C. Eisdorfer and M.P. Lawton (Eds.), The Psychology of Adult Development and Aging. Washington: American Psychological Association, 1973, pp. 343-377.

61. Wilder, D., Gurland, B.J., and Bennett, R. The chronicity of depression among the elderly. In: L. Erlenmeyer-Kimling, B. Dohrenwend, N. Miller (Eds.), Life Span Research on the Prediction of Psychopathology. Columbia University (in press).

62. Gurland, B.J. and Toner, J. Differentiating dementia from non-dementing conditions. In: R. Mayeux (Ed.), The Dementias. New York: Raven Press (in press).

63. Gurland, B.J. and Cross, P.S. Suicide among the elderly. The Acting-Out Elderly. Haworth Press (in press).

64. Challop, J., McCarthy, M., and Golden, R. Reliability and effects of training on rater's recognition of depression and dementia in elderly patients. Unpublished manuscript, 1982 (available from authors).

65. Gurland, B.J. A model for differential diagnosis of disturbed behavior in the elderly. Unpublished manuscript, 1982 (available from authors).

Other References

66. Kramer, M., Rosen, B., and Willis, E. Definitions and distribution of mental disorders in a racist society. In: Charles V. Willie et al. (Eds.), Racism and Mental Health. Pittsburgh: University of Pittsburgh Press, 1973, pp. 353-459.

67. Leighton, A. et al. Psychiatric disorder among the Yoruba: A report from the Cornell-Aro Mental Health Research Project in Western Region Nigeria. Ithaca, New York: Cornell University Press, 1963.

68. Bourestom, N. Evaluation of mental heath programs for the aged. Aging & Human Development, 1, pp. 187-219, 1970.

69. Elliot, J. Coatbridge: A survey into the needs of the elderly. Coatbridge, Scotland: Department of Social Work (Survey 1968-1969).

70. Sainsbury, P. Principles and Methods in Evaluating Community Psychiatric Services. Paper presented at Eighth International Congress of Gerontology, Washington, D.C., 1969.

71. Bennett, R. Social context - a neglected variable in research on aging. Aging & Human Development, 1, pp. 97-116, 1970.

72. Bennett, R. Community Mental Health Programs, with Specific Reference to Those Serving the Aged. Paper presented at Gerontological Society Institute, Ashville, North Carolina, 1971.

73. Hoenig, T. and Hamilton, M. Extramural care and the elderly. British Journal of Psychiatry, 113, pp. 435-443, 1967.

74. Kay, D.W.K., Beamish, P., and Roth, M. Old age mental disorders in Newcastle-upon-Tyne: Part I. A study of prevalence. British Journal of Psychiatry, 110, pp. 146-158, 1964.

75. Kramer, M., Taube, C., and Starr, S. Patterns of use of psychiatric facilitites by the aged: Current status, trends and implication. Psychiatric Research Reports, 23, 1968.

76. Lowther, C.P., MacLeod, R.D.M., and Williamson, J. Evaluation and early diagnostic services for the elderly. British Medical Journal, 3, pp. 275-277, 1970.

77. U.S. Department of Health, Education and Welfare. Public Health Service, Series 10, Number 70. Age Patterns in Medical Care, Illness and Disability, United States, 1968-1969.

78. Essen-Moller, E., Larsson, H., Uddenberg, C.E., and White, G. Individual traits and morbidity in a Swedish rural population. Acta Psychiatrica Scandinavica, Supplement 100, 1956.

79. New York State Department of Mental Hygiene, Mental Health Research Unit, A Mental Health Survey of Older People, Utica, New York: State Hospitals Press, 1960.

80. Primrose, E.J.R. Psychological Illness: A Community Study. Chicago: Charles C. Thomas, 1962.

81. Sheldon, J.H. The Social Medicine of Old Age: Report of an Enquiry in Wolverhampton. London: Oxford University Press, 1948.

82. Lowenthal, M.F., Berkman, P. and Associates. Aging and Mental Disorder in San Francisco. San Francisco: Jossey Bass, 1967.

83. Simon, A. and Neal, M.W. Patterns of geriatric mental illness. In: R.H. Williams, C. Tibbitts, and W. Donahue (Eds.), Processes of Aging. New York: Atherton Press, 1963.

84. Department of Health and Social Security. Psychiatric Hospitals and Units in England and Wales, Statistical Report Series, No. 12, Her Majesty's Stationery Office, London, 1969.

85. Kramer, M. and Taube, C. The Role of a National Statistics Program in the Planning of Community Psychiatric Services in the United States. Paper presented at Second World Psychiatric Association, Mannheim, West Germany, July, 1972.

86. Brotman, H.E. Income and poverty in the older population in 1975. The Gerontologist, 17, pp. 23-26, 1977.

87. Butler, R.N. Why Survive? On Being Old in America. New York: Harper and Row Publishers, 1975.

88. Shepherd, M., Cooper, B., Brown, A.C., and Kalton, G. Psychiatric Illness in General Practice. London: Oxford University Press, 1966.

89. Deming, Edwards, W. Uncertainties not attributable to sampling. In: Sample Design in Business Research, Ch. 5. New York: Wiley, 1960.

90. Deming, E.W. Statistical Theory of Optimum Allocation. Unpublished manuscript, 1975 (available from author).

91. Shanas, E., Townsend, P., Widderburn, D., Friss, H., Milhoj, D., and Stehouwer, J. Old People in Three Industrial Societies. New York: Atherton Press, 1968, p. 72.

92. Neugarten, B. Age groups in American society and the rise of the young-old. Ann. Am. Acad., September 1974, pp. 187-198.

93. U.S. Department of Health, Education and Welfare, P.H.S. Series 3, No. 3. Changes in Mortality Trends in England and Wales, 1931-1961.

94. U.S. Department of Health, Education and Welfare, P.H.S., Vol. II, Section 5. Vital Statistics of the United States, 1975, Life Tables.

95. U.S. Department of Commerce, Bureau of the Census, Marital Status and Living Arrangements, March 1974. Current Population Reports, Series P20, No. 271, October 1974.

96. U.N. Demographic Yearbook, 1973. United Nations, New York.

97. Deming, E.W. A cautionary note on the interpretation of survey data. Unpublished manuscript, 1965 (available from authors).

98. Siegel, S. Non-parametric Statistics for the Behavioral Sciences. New York: McGraw Hill, 1956.

99. The described material is available from authors, Dr. B.J. Gurland, Center for Geriatrics and Gerontology, 100 Haven Avenue, Tower III, 29-F, New York, New York 10032.

100. World Health Organization. International Classification of Diseases, 9th Edition, Geneva, Switzerland, 1975.

101. Kral, W.A. Senescent forgetfulness: Benign and malignant. Canadian Medical Association Journal (Toronto) 86, 257-260, 1962.

102. Pfeiffer, E. A short portable mental status questionnaire for the assessment of organic brain deficit in elderly patients. Journal of the American Geriatrics Society, 23, 1975.

103. Cronbach, L. Coefficient alpha and the international structure of tests. Psychometrics, 16, pp. 297-334, 1951.

104. Birkett, D.P., Gurland, B.J., Dean, L.L., and Wilder, D. Comparison of drug use by the elderly in New York and London. Unpublished manuscript, 1981 (available from authors).

105. Erdos, N. and Vernon, P. The assessment of the need for community based care for the elderly in Northeastern New York State. Final Report, 1982.

106. Wilder, D. The role of the current delivery system in the care of the chronic dependent elderly in New York State. Final Report, 1982.

107. Kemp, B., Plopper, M., and Lopez, W. Assessment of the health status, rehabilitation of the needs and barriers to health utilization among older Hispanics of Los Angeles. Final Report, 1982.

108. Cohen, C. and Sokolvsky, J. Social engagement versus isolation: The case of the aged in SRO hotels. The Gerontologist, 1980, 20(1), pp. 36-44.